HOW YOU'RE MEANT TO EAT

*A Complete Guide to Awaken Your Intuition
for a Seamless, Guilt-Free Eating Experience*

Avishek Saha

How You're Meant to Eat: A Complete Guide to Awaken Your Intuition for a Seamless and Guilt-Free Eating Experience. Avishek Saha.

Cover Design: Andie at 100covers.com

ISBN: 978-1-985758-41-4 (print)

Acknowledgements

Thank you for your interest in this book. You will soon discover my motivations for writing it, and my own evolving journey in connecting to my food. After a few years of intense restrictive dieting, I discovered two writers who helped me reconnect to my intuition and discover a common-sense approach to food. These writers were Matt Stone of 180degreehealth and Dr. Steven Bratman, the man who first coined the term "orthorexia," an unhealthy obsession with eating healthfully. I'm indebted to both of them, for their works helped me completely shift from a disordered approach to food to one embracing balance and overall health, rather than body fat or any other goal that tends to take the health enthusiast down a dark rabbit hole.

I thank my mother and father, for giving me the tools I needed to mature and develop a critical mind. I thank Dr. Doug Hanes of the National University of Natural Medicine, for showing me what humility and patience in science looks like, and for working closely with me in developing my research project, which unfortunately was never finished due to an unexpected closure of the laboratory and my decision to leave my master's program. Although I am no longer in the world of academia, my experience there was a privilege and taught me important lessons on critical thinking and patience.

I thank everyone who has left an encouraging comment on any of my content online—you keep me fueled. I like the negative comments too; as you may be aware, I promote brutal honesty and truth in my writing, and I hope for the same from readers, as it always leads to growth (unless you're a snowflake millennial). Lastly, I thank you, for investing in an idea that is unconventional and contrary to the norm, but which has the power to answer many of your health questions (and I want you to tell me how it works out for you).

Disclaimer and Disclosures

The information contained in this book is not a substitute for medical advice from a licensed physician or healthcare practitioner. The opinions shared throughout the book are for informative and educational purposes only. If you have medical concerns, consult with your physician.

To Lindsay
An anorexic who was never cured

Contents

Preface: Chapter Descriptions and Tips on Reading for Best Results

WHEN I SET OUT TO write this book, it started as a small project. It was just going to be a short guide. But as I wrote, I realized there was an important message I wanted to share with readers—a message developed from almost a decade of experience. This message is about connection—connection to nature. Initially, this book was meant for those recovering from eating disorders, as that's the crowd the concept of intuitive eating presently caters to.

But as I wrote about intuition and reminisced upon the times where it was woefully absent in my life, I realized that this book has a much broader focus, and thus, may be helpful to anyone remotely interested in what to eat, in addition to those who've had similar experiences as me in rabidly attempting a variety of diets. The idea of intuiting what to eat is not just for those with eating disorders, it is helpful for anyone who has become disconnected from a process we've relied on ever since we began walking on this Earth (estimated to be about a gazillion people).

If you have an illness, this book isn't designed to give you answers on its treatment. This book is about an innate process that's missing from our lives. Once you learn to implement it, you may find an answer to your dietary questions, but do not expect a complex illness to be healed from following any of the advice in this book. This also isn't a weight loss book. This clarification needs to be made because people often ask me medical questions, since I was in medical school once.

Based on what your interests are, I have some suggestions on how to read this book. If you are a general health enthusiast who wants to learn more about nutrition, you should read the book from start to finish. If you are recovering from an eating disorder, it's acceptable to start with part II, although you should still read the book from start to finish as there are two exercises in part I that may benefit you.

Exercises are scattered throughout the book, and they're designed to build upon each other. This book is a guide as well as a program. Thus, when you come upon the exercises, I strongly recommend you perform the exercise right then and there. Set a time to complete it in the near future if you cannot make that possible.

The following is a summary of each chapter. If any one in particular calls to you, feel free to skip ahead using the table of contents. Chapters 1 and 2 comprise part I, and attempt to establish why eating intuitively is desperately needed and can solve the common issues encountered with its converse (logical eating, the norm). The exercises in part I are very gentle and designed to start reviving your intuition.

Following chapter 2 is part II, which explains how intuition works. In chapter 3, we define what intuition is. In chapter 4, I recount the dietary experiments that have led me to embrace intuition in all aspects of my life presently. Chapter 5 discusses the several factors blocking people's intuition especially in understanding food. The two exercises in this section are designed to unblock intuition.

Part III outlines the methods to the *HYMTE* approach and starts with chapter 6, a discussion on hunger. Chapter 7 explains the steps to the *HYMTE* approach and is highly instructional, detailed, and contains four different exercises. In chapter 8, I discuss how to make sense of the intuitive information you'll receive about what foods to eat.

In chapter 9, I share two suggested plans to follow with instructions on how often to perform each of the exercises. The first plan is for those who have a history of chronic dieting and the second is for the general health enthusiast who has not burdened his or her body with years of dieting in the past. Chapter 10 is a conclusion, after which you'll find some references.

1:
Introduction—Digesting Health Information in Modern Times

My point is not to suggest that America isn't a wonderful country with our own rich history of cuisine. My point is that we're out of touch with our roots. That disconnection is the biggest reason why we have bookshelves full of conflicting nutritional advice.
—CATHERINE SHANAHAN, M.D.

THE ABUNDANCE OF INFORMATION at our fingertips about bone broth, insect proteins, and magical berries in the rainforest has massively improved our health, right? No. But what it has led to is a lot of confusion, failed attempts at weight loss, and attempts at "biohacking" our brains. Biohackers have been around since the origins of pharmaceutical medicines, but terms like those are excellent for deceiving those health fanatics who think they're onto something new.

What we have indeed accomplished is ingesting more types of strange compounds isolated from foods and "superfoods" than any human has in their evolutionary past. Some people even take over one hundred pills a day of various mineral, vitamin, and/or herb combinations to extend life, prevent disease, and maintain a healthy sex drive (the last one is crucial because it sells).

Compared to say living in Africa in 5,000 B.C. and eating wholesome meals with wild foods, it should in theory be even healthier to drink wheatgrass every day because—insert interesting sales pitch or scientific backing here—and take collagen supplements with lemon water each day for breakfast, right before intermittent fasting, and— well, you get my point. We have a lot of books, supplements, and ideas available to us that would have never been in our consciousness before the internet.

How much is this helping us, if at all? Are the health-conscious people doing better than they would, say, 5,000 years ago without collagen supplements, while living a simpler life (barring the possibility that they were eating more nutrient-dense food)? If you're a health fanatic, you will excitedly nod your head yes. "Of course! My wheatgrass is amazing! Without it, I'd have no energy to go to work, play with my kids, and—oh yea, I even healed my itchy anus with it!"

It would suck to admit that our beliefs and practices aren't serving us. It's how products which don't help the consumer stay on the market for longer. I'm all for natural medicines, food as medicine, and supplementation. But the claims that are often made to sell health products trick us, even if they seem to be backed up by "science."

If you found out that the benefits of wheatgrass were based on just hype, you'd feel scammed. Initially, you would defend your beliefs strongly, but after understanding that perhaps you did exaggerate how it helped your itchy anus, you'd see that you could obtain energy to go to work and play with your kids in many other ways. The wheatgrass was exciting, and that's it. It may have had some benefits, but it wasn't as amazing as you thought.

There are many professional scammers today who make claims surrounding "turbocharging your metabolism" sound very appealing, but ultimately deliver something that doesn't hold much promise at all for helping the consumer. They can go to such a degree in promoting a product with incorrect ideas that they make a compromise on ethics. For example, one famous doctor you may have heard of once claimed that eating more fiber could help detoxify the estrogen in women's blood that contributes to the pear-shaped phenotype a lot of women have. That's not even remotely true. There's a difference between explaining something to patients succinctly so they can better understand it and making claims that simply aren't true just to excite them about your services and ideas.

Science is often used as a marketing technique for scams of this nature. The "science" is used to justify the product, but doesn't usually ever do so directly in the form of a clinical trial. What I've seen to be the case countless times is that the claim was based off just one laboratory study, involving cell cultures or animals—this describes most bodybuilding supplements on the market. These studies usually can't lend much support to the idea of a human, rather than a cell culture, benefiting from that supplement. But it doesn't matter. It's about hype, and the science is only important in amplifying hype, the crucial selling sauce.

But even if the claims are based off of a clinical trial of sorts, the supplement company often funded the trial. Conflicts of interest thus weaken the study's findings, even if it's a great product. If it helps people, that's wonderful. But the problem here, and the raison d'être for this book, is that this exact type of agenda-promoting science is what makes its way into the layman's consciousness regarding health. Much of what we think we know about health comes from flawed and biased research that is never interpreted right by the media. The goal of the media is to obtain views; they won't report the boring facts as much as create sensational headlines.

When we consequently construct a dietary paradigm from sensationalism, we end up with the health predicament we're in today: utterly confused despite information spilling out from our brains. Surely, when we think of what's healthy, or what's not healthy, we'd like to think, just like we did about wheatgrass, that the science our conclusions are based off of are sound! Telling ourselves we are wrong requires humility, which the vast majority of people resist initially.

For some in fact, admitting wrongs is simply unfathomable; and if that's you, you will not find this book pleasurable to read. Eating intuitively according to the *HYMTE* approach requires you to change your opinions based on the information your body gives you, which could change after you finish reading this paragraph. Unlike a predictable meal-plan, your body is not predictable. The weather is not always predictable. Your mood isn't predictable. Why should your diet be then? Nature is crazy! There is no room in intuitive eating for your preconceived notions about what to eat to dictate what you eat.

Further, intuitive eating goes beyond food; the techniques outlined in this book to enhance your intuition can be used to improve your decision-making process in all areas of life. With fitness for example, you may think there is solid science that high-intensity interval training (HIIT), which was all the rage years ago, helps you burn more fat than slow-steady state cardio. Perhaps you used to frequently go hiking—not as a workout per se—but just to wind down and relax. Then, you suddenly read the latest research on HIIT, which made slow-steady state cardio look worthless. Now you're thinking: "Oh gosh! I just read that steady-state cardio makes you hungrier and can cause weight gain! I must stop hiking, start HIIT, and join a CrossFit gym now. Oh well. Bye nature!"

But if you apply your intuition to this scenario, you'll take the science with a grain of salt, and before jumping to any conclusions, will ask your body for feedback. You will then try HIIT a few times, and check in with yourself to understand how you feel. And from there, you'll either add HIIT to your life if you find it valuable, or just hike as you used to. Perhaps you already did some HIIT when you hiked, because intuitively, you found that you enjoyed doing some short sprints on certain stretches of the hike.

I've jumped on many bandwagons, including HIIT, each time developing an intense excitement toward the idea. This is a common scenario and I overhear conversations about it frequently. One conversation on a bus went like this: "My nutrition professor talked about the ketogenic diet today. Half the class switched to a low-carbohydrate diet overnight!" I was compelled to say something but I honor that people have their own journey, and most people are able to use their intuition to discard what doesn't work.

Unfortunately, there are some people who decide to devote themselves to the process, and stay low-carb despite signs that their health isn't ideal anymore. There is a strong belief system supporting their views and to challenge that belief system would be undoing the learning they've spent months on via research and experimentation.

I've had to let go of many beliefs I invested considerable time and energy in applying to my life just to come to terms with the mismatch between experience and research. What is presented to you in this book is essentially a culmination of those experiences: a method of eating that is designed to give you an understanding of food and your own body that is fad-proof. After you read this work, you'll know how to identify a new concept in health and decide whether or not it truly works for your body. Instead of *just* following the latest research, you will follow your body too. And my ultimate aim is that you'll be able to eat without as much confusion.

In the next chapter we will explore a few important topics in nutrition science to illustrate the problems with relying on it exclusively, and why there is a consequent need to eat intuitively. I do not mean to suggest that research is inherently bad. I love research. But for a variety of reasons that we will explore, its quest to find truth can become diluted, leading to wrong conclusions about health. Although nutrition research can help us understand what to eat, it has weaknesses, and we can learn from them to better inform our health decisions.

Intuition-Building Exercise #1: Walking Meditation in Nature

But before that it's time for your first exercise to build, unlock, and enhance your intuition. There will be many more scattered throughout this book, and I recommend performing them as soon as possible. This one is about connecting to nature. Identify a natural spot near you and spend at least one hour in that spot with nothing other than yourself. The instructions are to simply spend time in this environment in observation. No phones, no friends, or books even are allowed. Dogs are okay, unless they're overly distracting.

The purpose of this exercise is to connect your primal mind to the natural environment, with *nothing* in-between. Phones help us connect with other people. You can take a nice picture with it, and send it to your friends, telling them you were in nature. But you're not fully connecting intimately with nature when you do this.

Similarly, you could go to this spot with your friends and talk so much that you never pay attention to your surroundings. Not acceptable here. This is an exercise, and that's why we need to be extreme for at least one hour. You simply will not understand your intuition without connecting to nature. People who lived in the

Paleolithic era did it after all. They were so smart they got a diet named after them that was completely unrelated to the diet they were actually on. (If they saw what the paleo diet was now they might even get offended).

So what do I mean by a natural spot? Ideally it is a place slightly off the grid with no cellular service—a forest of some kind. A beach is also a great idea. If you are too far away from places like this, find a trail nearby that has a lot of nature in it. The paths should ideally be dirt paths and everywhere you look you should see nature. The worst-case scenario is an urban environment that has some trees and is meant to be somewhat natural. There are studies however showing that that even spending time in these man-made environments can reduce stress, although never as much as the most natural environments.[1]

As you spend time in this environment, observe your surroundings. Take in the sights and smells. Listen. Walk around, sit, crawl, and move in whichever way you'd like. *Become one with this environment.*

Then, imagine that you are looking for food and start thinking about what you'd want to eat as if the apocalypse came early and there were no more grocery stores. You don't have to come up with an exact answer to this. Just entertain the notion that you are fully connected to your primal mind and know how to hunt and gather in any natural setting. Observe everything around you and enjoy the experience.

From doing this exercise you will start activating a part of you that has been buried from living a modern life, and that is your intuition. All of this will be explained in future chapters.

If you don't live near a natural environment and opt for something closer to you, spend at least an hour there walking, sitting, and/or meditating. If you choose to go for a hike or walk along the beach, spend more than an hour there. Let your brain be soothed, and practice connecting to your environment like the human that you are. And I would suggest avoiding the temptation to write everything down and process it logically. If you come from a logical background, it is even more important that you avoid this. If you are artistically-inclined, then it is okay to write a few things down, as you likely won't be perpetuating logic-dominance (we will discuss why this is important in part II). This exercise is all about experience.

What are you waiting for? Take a break, and come back once your mind has absorbed nature's sights, sounds, and smells. Or, if you want to continue reading, set a time on your calendar to follow through with this exercise. But if you're a chronic procrastinator like me, make sure you do it soon, otherwise you'll forget!

PART I

SCIENCE VS. INTUITION—BALANCING OUR APPROACH TO FOOD

Although we perceive science as an ultimate truth, science is finally just a story, told in installments.

—LYNNE MCTAGGART

2:

Understanding Nutrition Science, Discarding It, and Then Replacing It with Intuition

And certainly, we should take care not to make the intellect our god; it has, of course, powerful muscles, but no personality. It cannot lead, it can only serve; and it is not fastidious in its choices of a leader. This characteristic is reflected in the qualities of its priests, the intellectuals. The intellect has a sharp eye for methods and tools, but is blind to ends and values. So it is no wonder that this fatal blindness is handed from old to young and today involves a whole generation.

—ALBERT EINSTEIN

SCIENCE CAN BE VERY exciting. And that makes it a great tool for marketing a product. The science generally enhances the fervor people will develop for a fad diet or a seemingly new idea. But it's not the findings that excite us. It's the *implications* it has. Hope. Sometimes, this sentiment grows so strong it mutates into a disease characterized by religion-like fervor. That's what I experienced first-hand within the various dietary ideologies I subscribed to in the past. It is human nature and it will never change.

What we can change, and what I have been forced to change over the years, is our understanding of nutrition science. What role does it play in informing our health practices? Where does funding for nutrition research come from and what are the implications of this? What is and isn't studied in a scientific experiment or clinical trial? What can we accurately conclude from the research we read? Let's attempt to answer these questions by examining several cases.

First, consider Soylent, a food-product designed to save time. It contains everything we need, *in theory*, based on nutrition science.[2] It has vitamins, minerals, proteins, fats, carbohydrates, etc. These are logical arguments, which are the mainstay of any food's health benefits.

But why would most of us choose against drinking Soylent daily to support our metabolic needs? Simply because it's non-intuitive to drink your food every day without enjoying its smells, tastes, and textures. This product doesn't have the variety of tastes that a varied diet has. But in theory, Soylent still contains all the nutrients that we need to function properly. From an intuitive perspective however (which entails the experience of food and other factors we will discuss in parts II and III), it's lacking in most ways I can think of.

The disciplines of chemistry, biochemistry, physics, and biology, among others, have revealed to us what is in our foodstuffs, and they certainly play a vital role in elucidating our bodies' requirements. But do we *need* them to know how to eat healthfully? Are the discoveries about food that have been made by these disciplines enabling us to eat more healthfully than we did in our evolutionary past, or compared to people with a strong cultural background where food is an important component?

The answer is no. Sometimes scientists and our Western culture seems to act as if we have it all figured out and are coming up with new ideas that have never been figured out before. This type of thinking doesn't give enough credence to brilliant ideas that come from other cultures with a different, and difficult-to-translate, worldview.

Consider an ancient system of healing known as Traditional Chinese medicine (TCM), dating back to several thousand years BCE. Chemistry wasn't around then. The Chinese doctors who came up with this system did not think of their foods as proteins, carbohydrates, or fats. To them food contained a mix of different energies, qualities, and other properties described simply as hot, cold, bitter, dry, astringent, damp, and in many other ways. Nutrition science defines energy as kilocalories. In contrast, in TCM, energy is a metaphor, and subsequently, everything has an energy. For the chronic and confused dieter, I recommend forgetting all of what science has taught us and start fresh, as if we are living in pre-modern times.

I do not intend to suggest we get rid of science completely in our discussions of health; we need to form a healthy relationship with it. And for that reason, we must detach from it temporarily. I believe this will help us connect to food as pre-modern humans did. Once this is established, it will be productive again to implement science in our understanding of food. But for now, even a concept like "energy" which has a precise definition must be forgotten and instead replaced with the metaphorical use of word, which will be expounded upon in chapter 7, where we discuss the *HYMTE* approach.

Science, as much as I enjoy reading it, does disconnect us from nature and intuition. From my experience within the schooling system, no matter what the discipline is, adopting a scientific approach to studying nature strips away the innate and primal aspect to *living* in nature. It just can't be mimicked in the classroom. To study nature scientifically, we must apply some degree of separation. We must isolate something and observe it in a controlled setting to understand how it works—or so we're told.

For example, once I studied abroad in Peru while at the University of Maryland, to study medicinal plants of the Amazon rainforest. Boats took us to our lodging, off the grid. The experience was intensely calming to my central nervous system. Looking across the Amazon river at the dense tropical foliage, while traveling to my destination on boat was a truly blissful experience. I realized I had been living in a highly stimulated state for quite some time.

One day, as we discussed medicinal plants, the advisor of the trip made this comment: "most of the medicinal plants in the Amazon are unknown; there could be a billion-dollar cure here!" I was perplexed. I thought I went there to study medicinal plants, but being quite naïve at the time, I didn't realize that a typical college education in the United States places greater emphasis on teaching students how to discover a lucrative new drug that only marginally helps people over teaching herbal medicine, a practice reserved for "charlatans," as the mainstream medical world would have it. This was one of the first signs I failed to notice with my intuition that school wasn't going to give me the education I was looking for. My advisor and I had completely different interests.

Although my father works in drug discovery, for whatever reason (I'll blame it on the stars), I became passionate about studying all things "natural." I realized there was knowledge that just wasn't taught in schools, and moreover, was ostracized and ridiculed. It's evident now that this attitude towards "complementary" and "alternative" medicines was largely engineered by a system that was set up to squelch it over a century ago.

I thus became determined to discover that knowledge for myself, and I stupidly thought that going on a study abroad trip was going to help me do this. Although my exposure to the rainforest and meeting Jim Duke, a renown ethnobotanist, was a transformational experience,

I became slightly unnerved that something major seemed to be missing from the "science" that was so highly regarded throughout my entire time in school.

Puzzle Pieces

The type of science I refer to is the science I've spent a lot of time trying to pack into my short-term memory. It's also a lot like doing a sudoku puzzle. This type of science is about finding puzzle pieces and putting them together, to construct a theory about how the universe works. This puzzle is separate and divisible, and when the puzzle is our own bodies, the body is viewed as a machine—the sum of its parts. Descartes and Newton among others played a strong role in creating this type of thinking in the West.

Although putting puzzle pieces together is fun for some (I only like it in a metaphorical sense, whereas, actual puzzles with literal puzzle pieces bore me) in medicine, nutrition, and biological sciences, this thinking can lead to incorrect conclusions about how things work much of the time. A recent experience in medical school (before I left) confirmed these thoughts. I saw just how mistaken even a licensed physician can be when applying nutrition research to clinical practice.

In my first clinical rotation, I saw a patient one day who we diagnosed with iron-deficiency anemia. She was vegetarian, but knowing that she was Mexican and Mexicans love red meat, I figured I'd ask her if she was open to adding it to her diet. She said yes. But as a secondary on that shift (the student who takes vital signs but mostly observes) my power to dictate what was prescribed was limited. My job was to take vitals and clean up; it was not to share too many of my opinions (although that should have been encouraged as much as possible, but sadly, the art of discussion is a lost one in many academic institutions). The best I could do to truly help patients in that role was to attempt starting a conversation and just see where it went.

Since arrogance is quite common in the medical field, it's often difficult when you're a student to have a voice. People like to think they know what they're doing and it's another unfortunate mindset endemic to the healthcare profession. Not only are they trained to dismiss thousands of years of traditional wisdom on healing, they often think they know much more than they actually do. And much of that knowledge is incomplete because it's not based on intuition; applying intuition to healthcare is difficult, and likely a bit too abstract to be taken seriously.

I shared my thoughts with the primary. She kept insisting on iron supplementation, because the endless memorizing required to pass tests in medical school taught her to separate things into their parts and add up the parts that mattered. The attending physician on that shift also favored iron supplementation. This was at a naturopathic medical school, a place I enrolled in hoping to study natural medicines. Here, the idea of food as medicine is quite popular. It sounds great too, but often, something that sounds great doesn't work as great in practice. Unfortunately, food as medicine isn't profitable enough for it to become a regular part of a doctor's prescription.

Seeing the resistance to my ideas, I carefully framed my point of view, and eventually, the primary liked the idea so much she acted as if it were her own. Again, the arrogance made it difficult for her to ever express a genuine interest in the idea and acknowledge its merit. It was my goal to at least try my best to voice myself in a tactful way, because I wouldn't feel satisfied if I saw that patient go home with an iron supplement. I'm all for some supplementation to the diet, but when we choose supplementation over treating the root cause repeatedly, we're being lazy. Funnily, treating the root cause is one of the modern day naturopathic physician's mottos. It also sounds better than is practical.

Food *is* medicine, I thought, but why was it so hard to follow this simple idea in the clinic? Experiences like this one continued to have me question how intuition could be added to healthcare. I often felt like few others seemed interested in this endeavor, and I myself didn't have much of an idea how to apply intuition to practice. I slowly learned about the mess of insurance reimbursement, and I started to see that there were additional challenges no one told me about as a student that could influence a doctor's decisions. Ideas are great, but their implementation is what matters. Implementing abstract unproven ideas with little to no research dollars behind them simply doesn't have a future in healthcare.

In the conference room we discussed the case. What I heard next made me facepalm—mentally at least. "Let's prescribe some red meat with lemon," suggested the attending physician. I felt that I was near my quota for challenging people on that shift so I didn't say any more. This "naturopathic" clinic shift was very frustrating because something was always terribly wrong every week.

What this doctor recommended was based on "science" that was interpreted incorrectly. She was thinking about how red meat contains iron, lemons contain vitamin C, and there are studies showing that vitamin C enhances the absorption of iron. 1 + 1 = 2. Yay! Science. I love science. Well, it's not that simple.

The studies she was thinking of did not examine iron absorption after consumption of red meat with vitamin C. They looked at absorption of just one form of iron in the presence of ascorbic acid (Vitamin C). [3,4] They are two different scenarios entirely. Your reductionist brain may be thinking that if iron absorption is enhanced with vitamin C, why wouldn't it work with our food? What's the big deal Avishek? Why are you throwing a fit?

I'm not throwing a fit! OK fine—there are many reasons why I'm throwing a fit. One is that those studies used nonheme iron, whereas meat contains heme iron, the absorption of which is not enhanced with vitamin C. Secondly, what about the effect of all the other beneficial things in meat, like fat, protein, zinc, and antioxidants on the absorption of heme iron? I'd hypothesize that the whole food would improve iron absorption. And beyond that, what about the effect of the other components of a balanced *meal* containing red meat on the absorption of iron? Well, it seems that since before 1980 it was known that combining vegetable sources of nonheme iron failed to enhance iron absorption.[5] From that paper:

> Absorption therefore appears to be a property of the overall composition of the meal rather than of the single food item. These studies led to a very important observation. If a small quantity of soluble inorganic iron is added to a biosynthetically labeled vegetable food just before it is eaten, percentage absorption of the two forms of iron is nearly identical. The same is true of meals containing more than one vegetable food. Therefore it appears that when several foods are eaten together, nonheme iron destined for absorption behaves as if it were from a single common pool.

What the above quote essentially implies is that when synthetic iron is added to a food containing non-heme iron, absorption of iron is as if they were taken separately—in other words, there is no change. The effect isn't additive. They also point out: "heme iron absorption is relatively independent of other components of the meal; ascorbic acid has no effect." Recall that heme iron is the kind present in red meat. However, this study does not answer the questions I posed above, about how multiple foods together along with red meat together could influence how heme-iron is absorbed. I don't think it's very important.

Imagine something with me. Here is one isolated case of a well-intentioned prescription involving misinterpreted science. How many other cases like this do you think there are? And this case just involves misinterpreted research, as well as a lack of effort in reading the research. Doctors don't have a lot of time to read research. But aside from not reading the research, in those cases where research was discovered, how many other cases of bad advice is given to patients by doctors based on flawed, biased, *and* misinterpreted research?

Further, how much misinformation is spread by *other* healthcare practitioners like registered dietitians, nurse practitioners, physical therapists, and any other practitioners based on flawed, biased, and misinterpreted research? And lastly, how much misinformation is spread by the *media* with sensational headlines to readers who don't think twice about looking up the original source of the study, and secondly, don't have the background to understand *how* to interpret that research regardless?

If we quantified this as the total number of instances where these grievances occurred, I would estimate it to rival the United States' national debt.

Most anyone talking about science is misinformed until proven otherwise in my opinion, unless they clearly acknowledge that there is room for error—massive room. One statistician in fact, John Ionnidis, boldly asserts that most published research findings are false, due to a variety of biases, and the way most studies determine significance—a p-value of 0.05 (a completely arbitrary number). These results become even more problematic when paired with the small effect sizes research is often plagued by.[6] If he is even somewhat correct, then we must reconsider the science backing up our dietary beliefs and supplement regimens.

This doesn't mean we should give up on science. We should certainly try to understand research. But the vast majority of us are misinformed, and much of science is flawed, biased, agenda promoting, and on the other hand, is not even read. Yet, we base our conclusions off of it daily. Some studies are also more widely cited than others; most published research just sits on a dusty bookshelf somewhere and no one ever knows about it. After enough time has passed, it is completely forgotten, even if it was a well-designed study.

If we want to do our best to understand science, we must realize it will take work. And this is not going to be a popular option for most people who buy health products and read about health for fun. It's just too much work. But if science is truly interesting to you, I urge you to set the intention to get better at reading it. Create habits so that you read it regularly. Find open access journals and download some free PDF files and make time to read them. Slowly, but surely, the language of science will begin to make more sense.

But most importantly, we must understand the limitations of the research we read. We must see that the puzzle we're trying to construct is connected to another puzzle, which is connected to other puzzles, which connects to another galaxy of puzzles, instead of becoming overly excited by headlines that mistakenly report on one single study.

Thinking Holistically

When we start thinking holistically, in terms of meals and not just individual foods or constituents, adding vitamin C to iron seems so trivial—so disconnected. Perhaps seemingly trivial details can improve our lives. After all, we should not glorify holistic thinking as much as we've glorified reductionism. But after we accumulate enough puzzle pieces, we may ask ourselves if the plethora of details these pieces provide leads to better health. No, they don't, and we don't need them I've decided.

Although I do find the details fascinating, I'm now more fascinated by the whole. Imagining the "whole" in any instant seems to require a fundamentally different way of thinking and perceiving than what is generally taught to us in schools. Details may help inform the whole, but without the whole, we will forever be disconnected.

What can happen as a result of this disconnection is the completion of a puzzle with pieces that don't quite fit together. We then focus just on this puzzle and forget all the other ones we haven't completed yet. This incomplete puzzle is a diet—any diet. Then, we stick to a diet that makes sense based on the puzzle pieces, but on the whole is absurd and ill-equipped to produce good health. A fad. Fads are the brand-new box the puzzle game comes in. We focus on that puzzle alone, forget the rest, and then call it a day.

What most puzzles have in common is they isolate components of food, then reverse engineer a diet. Funnily enough, many engineers and mathematicians who dabble in the world of nutrition as a hobby are attracted to this type of thinking. But this is not how we're meant to eat. That doesn't mean it can't work. It just doesn't work too well on average, based on the plethora of dietary advice in existence that contradicts each other multiple times over and produces ill-health, which we rarely hear about because people want to hold on to the notion that their belief-system is a cure-all.

Now, meant is a strong word. Suggesting that we are meant to eat a certain way can make it seem as if other approaches do not work. Eating logically, and based off of "evidence," a buzzword, can sometimes produce great results. But it's not the way we've eaten for nearly all our existence as humans. Moreover, the concept of evidence-based medicine is a cultural paradigm, but not a truth-based one. Evidence in this paradigm, and as a buzzword, excludes all empirical data, subjective anecdotal experiences, even clinical experiences (unless published in a case report in which case they rank as the lowest quality of evidence) and purports that we must have a control group and an experimental group, otherwise we cannot learn anything about the universe. Those that hold knowledge must have a higher degree. This is completely false, and basing our diets off evidence within this paradigm is risky, naïve, and fallacious. It certainly is not how we are "meant" to eat, and this has broad implications.

The solution I propose to deal with this strange, modern predicament is to connect to nature and view food with a different lens than the type found within a microscope. Instead of isolating, let's see the whole. Instead of determining a food's chemical composition before attempting to understand its health benefits, let's think about its abstract qualities and what we desire from it intuitively. Let's *love* what we eat. Let's hate what we eat too, because that's a feeling, rather than a thought.

There are a myriad of other examples in nutrition where the science gets diluted and misinterpreted, separating us from our food, and resulting in unhelpful advice. In the next three examples, we will further investigate how relying on nutrition science alone can alienate us from our common sense and intuitive understanding of food. As you think about these examples, tune into how you feel about any foods or constituents being discussed. Ask yourself how you intuitively feel about its health benefits (in the case of curcumin next) or detriments (in the case of saturated fat), as you read the science on it.

Crazy for Curcumin

It is commonly believed that black pepper increases the absorption of turmeric (a root related to ginger that is commonly used in southeast Asian cooking). Google it. You'll find on the first page of Google many articles recommending the addition of black pepper to turmeric, to improve the medicinal properties of turmeric. One popular clickbait-type site says:

> ...combined with black pepper which offers its own set of benefits, turmeric works magic. Together, the black pepper-turmeric combo relieves pain, suppresses inflammation, helps lose weight, and prevents cancer.

Sounds to me as if they hired someone from Fiverr to write that, as most people on that site don't have the best grammar. The idea that black pepper enhances the absorption of turmeric has just as little evidence behind it as the assertion that eating lemons with meat will enhance iron absorption.

I argued on the train once with a crazy health-fanatic who clearly read little to no research explaining to me how grapeseed extract was a cure-all. I told him grapeseed is just "alright," unenthused. "There are a ton of compounds which do the same exact thing," I replied. The science creates hype, we forget what wasn't studied, and then end up glorifying a single compound, when the reality is we could find a plethora of other compounds that have similar medicinal actions, whether we're talking about quercetin, resveratrol, curcumin, berberine, or any other "active" ingredient.

He then switched the subject and ranted about black pepper increasing turmeric absorption, and I told him that there were simply no studies on this. They're on *curcumin* and black pepper absorption I pointed out (curcumin is the "active ingredient" in turmeric). I encouraged him to look up this fact, but as I attempted explaining how *interesting* this is instead of pretending I was trying to prove him wrong, he became frustrated and walked away. I'm used to that, especially in Portland where people are ultra-sensitive.

There were about six people sitting around us who seemed to be entertained by this debate; they congratulated me after the man walked away, as if I had won some sort of battle. If he wasn't so opinionated and attached to grapeseed extract, it wouldn't have seemed this way. Attachment is a very important intuition-blocking factor that we will get to in chapter 5.

Let's think about how science works in this example. *Why* would someone decide to conduct an experiment examining the effect of *curcumin bioavailability* from a *curcumin supplement* in the presence of black pepper, instead of conducting the same experiment with *turmeric*? Hmm... Well, curcumin isn't something we can extract readily in our kitchens. But as a supplement, it's something that can sell.

Turmeric supplements on the other hand make no sense. You can buy turmeric powder; why should we spend $30 a month for turmeric capsules when we can get the powder for much cheaper? I bet people would still swallow turmeric powder capsules not knowing any better, but curcumin still is a much more viable idea for a supplement. The next step now is to convince people that curcumin supplementation can lower their inflammation or solve other health issues more so than food alone.

All that's required now is a small trial of sorts observing the effect of taking a daily dose of curcumin, say 1500 mg, on inflammatory markers in patients with rheumatoid arthritis or some other inflammatory condition with an adequate control group for comparison. If curcumin successfully lowers markers of inflammation in the study's participants, doctors can then say that a preliminary trial supports the prescription of curcumin for the treatment of rheumatoid arthritis. It would most likely be preliminary trial here because studies on supplements don't get as much funding or go through as rigorous of a process as studies on new drugs. In fact, trials on supplements, which the FDA classifies as a food, are not permitted to ever become as large as the phase I-III trials drugs go through. The results of these preliminary trials are nothing more than "cute" to the medical world, as they are often underpowered and pale in comparison to drug research.

After the publication of trials like this, there is a press release. The news now carries the song of hope to the general public. Headlines read: "CURCUMIN LOWERS INFLAMMATION 25% WOW!" Manufacturers of curcumin supplements now can make bolder claims surrounding their product's efficacy, skirting around the FDA's limitations on making claims on the treatment of any disease (which is of course ridiculous).

And just like that, people become massively confused. They stock their shelves with the supplement, ingesting it daily. They forget about food's benefits. Food isn't exciting anymore. The $50 bottle of curcumin however—now that's all the rage.

When studies come out, we focus on what was seen and forget what wasn't seen. We have no idea if the curcumin supplement would be superior to food in reducing symptoms of rheumatoid arthritis in our hypothetical trial. All we know is that it's superior to a *control* condition, where subjects ingested a placebo pill.

One recent morning, I ate some eggs, stir-fried with kale, garlic, and one Thai green chili. I also made myself some caffeine-free chai (as I ran out of tea) with various spices. It's a meal with a mind-boggling number of interactions (which have not been studied). Pasture-raised eggs, cooked kale, garlic, the chili, cardamom, ginger, cinnamon, honey—can this combination of ingredients induce a health benefit as potent as the flashy ones offered by neatly labeled and packaged supplements such as curcumin? Yes. They absolutely can.

Certainly, curcumin has many studied benefits. But if we were to see those benefits in comparison to the fundamental factors that produce great health, I doubt it would look as exciting. Curcumin would seem unnecessary. Overkill. Overhyped. But fancy. As I mentioned in chapter 1, since we have a lack of connection to food, due to a loss of traditional wisdom and other factors, we often get more excited about products that we don't need to improve our health. How do you think meditating, eating food that's right for your body, exercising in moderation, practicing yoga, sleeping well every night, and obtaining adequate sunlight compare to a curcumin supplement? There isn't much comparison in my view. When we put things in context, step back, and understand how messages are advertised to us, we will become less confused about what to do.

The fact is that there are zero studies showing that black pepper enhances the absorption of *turmeric* (rather than curcumin). Just as there are numerous factors that produce good health, there are numerous constituents in turmeric aside from curcumin that have medicinal properties; yet, curcumin is throned as the "active" ingredient. I wonder how Indian people, who regularly cook with turmeric, feel about curcumin. I know what my grandmother would say that's for sure: "EAT FOOD BOY!" She would throw a bigger fit than me too surely.

Jim Duke, the ethnobotanist who created the Phytochemical and Ethnobotanical Databases as part of his work with the United States Department of Agriculture,[7] expressed to me firmly, but gently at his old age, that "there is no such thing as an active ingredient." Plants have thousands of compounds, and there are usually a few that synergize with the "active ingredient," which should be thought of more as the leader of the pack. Without the pack, it's simply not the same ingredient anymore.

Looking at James' ethnobotanical database, we can see that there are 267 identified constituents in all parts of the turmeric plant (*Curcuma longa*)[8] and 22 in just the root. One of the compounds in the root is 1,8-cineole, or eucalyptol, which as you may guess is found in eucalyptus. Others include ar-turmerone, beta-sitosterol, zingiberene (found in ginger), stigmasterol, salicylates, and several other kinds of curcuminoids. All of these compounds are anti-inflammatory, and I would surmise synergize with curcumin and its metabolites once ingested.

Do you think that curcumin now is really as wonderful as everyone says it is? The idea of all these compounds working together is far more interesting to me than the effects of curcumin alone. I could bore you with another several pages summarizing studies of each of these individual compounds in turmeric root but I hope you get the point, which is that many of the popular health ideas circulating in our consciousness come to us with a purpose: to sell, and this requires that we maintain a narrow field of vision. The barrage of ideas on the health benefits of individual things can produce a deficiency in common sense, intuition, and the big picture among those who internalize the information.

The experiments on curcumin don't benefit us as much as they benefit those turning it into a supplement. I'm not against that by any means. This is just an expected side effect of capitalism. What I'm attempting to show you is that science and business go hand in hand. Science, as objective as you think it might be, is often performed to benefit some industry, some product, or some business. In the world of nutrition science and medical research, this is often required. And thus, drawing conclusions about what you put into your body from "science" alone is a big mistake. We don't need that sort of science to understand how to eat healthfully.

The Healthy Eating Index (HEI)

Based on science again, the United States Department of Agriculture devised the healthy eating index (HEI),[9] a tool for assessing the healthiness of a diet for research purposes. Diets are given a score from 0-100 based on the amount of ten factors in the diet: fruits, vegetables, grains, milk, meat, total fat, saturated fat, cholesterol, sodium, and overall variety. There are ten maximum achievable points in each category. For total fat, saturated fat, cholesterol, and sodium, obtaining less than the maximum recommended amount in your diet gives you a score of 10.

Based on the HEI, a raw food diet automatically gifts you 40 points. This diet involves consuming only uncooked plant foods: fruits, vegetables, nuts, and seeds. Like Soylent, this sounds unappealing to sane folk. But those who are insane (like I was) convince themselves that the diet is an excellent recipe for health. They've adopted a strong belief system, and completely abandoned their intuition. And as a result, they've unfortunately chosen a path to ill health.

The raw food diet surely is not varied, and thus it wouldn't receive a high score under that category in the HEI. But overall, it could easily achieve a score above 60, which is far more than it should get based on how terrible it is for health. Having been on that diet for thirteen months, I am well aware that it is not a balanced diet nor one that produces anything but deficiency. But when we use the HEI, we see that the raw food diet could receive a higher score than a "standard American diet" (SAD).

The SAD has been universally labeled as a terrible diet for our health, for relying on agricultural methods that may not be sustainable, and for promoting the consumption of foods that aren't actually foods, but food-like products—foods many of us grew up with. These foods can be addicting, low in nutrition, and high in refined sugar. They are certainly a recipe for poor health down the line for most people. Thus, it's surprising to think that a raw food diet could be worse than the SAD.

Imagine however eating only fruits and vegetables with nuts and seeds every day for an extended period of time. There would be a lot of chewing. The food wouldn't be warm. The raw food diet is almost the opposite of the SAD in a sense. The SAD is weight-promoting, and the raw food diet is weight-loss promoting, but not necessarily in a healthy way. The raw food diet contains very little protein or fats, vitamin B12, and many other nutrients, and thus the weight loss if sustained long term could become a sign of malnourishment.

So how is it possible that in the HEI the raw food diet could receive far more points than the standard American diet, despite also producing poor health? One reason is because the studies the HEI is based off of don't evaluate food **synergy**, something that happens every time you eat, taste, and smell food. This *entire time* we've been studying food in a way that does not mimic how we prepare and consume it. We have asked questions about single foods and our health, like meat, or vegetables, or fruit, but have we asked a question such as: "what is the effect of eating high quality animal products *with* some vegetables, *with* some fruits, *with* some spices on our health?"

"Wait, isn't that the Mediterranean diet?" I wish, but that diet has been reduced to its parts so much that it does not resemble the type of balanced diet people in that part of the world consume. So not quite, and thus, when we sum up the parts, the raw food diet actually looks pretty good. From a holistic perspective however, it's lacking in warm foods, animal foods, fats, proteins, and a variety of tastes, all of which the standard American diet is undoubtedly too rich in. When we start seeing the whole, we will forget about the individual details, and instead, consider how we feel overall from any assortment of foods.

Have we even considered how the activities surrounding eating influence our health? This is also missing from the HEI, as well as most discussions on food that take place. How do you think socializing while eating, a common scenario, influences health? How does socializing with a friend while eating in a private residence compare to socializing at a corporate dinner where you're trying to climb the ladder? The latter situation is more stressful for most people and thus is less healthy (most likely) than socializing in a lower-pressure and more comfortable setting. The blood is just not flowing to the right places for optimal digestion when you're under pressure.

Experiences like this surrounding the eating of food can confer health benefits or detriments beyond the nature of what is eaten. Thus, the health fanatic who is constantly worrying about what to eat may be unhealthy due to high amounts of stress. It's hard to study such a complex interplay of factors in a controlled scientific setting, but I believe we can figure much of it out by trusting our gut.

As an example, imagine eating a plain hard-boiled egg, without any spices, vegetables, or sauces. Take a bite (mentally). How does it make you feel? Remember that. Now, add a dash of black pepper. Then, add some salt. Add ketchup, if you like ketchup. Note the difference in qualities of each bite, as well as their interactions, at each step, as well as noting how you feel about it.

If you're like me, the plain, hard-boiled egg just isn't as appetizing as the hard-boiled egg with some added flavors to it, like salt, pepper, and a little ketchup. The health implications of this aren't well known scientifically. The way the salt makes you feel isn't a quantifiable measure that is generally studied. Salt, or sodium chloride, has clear actions in the human body, and is certainly stress-relieving, but is it necessary to know the exact details to make you feel more comfortable about what you're eating anyway?

If you come from a background of disordered eating habits, or perfectionistic dieting, then perhaps you'd like to know all those details. What I'm telling you in this book is that the feeling you get itself is knowledge. Before I ate based on feelings, I ate relatively plain meals, low in sodium, sugar, and refined carbohydrate. But I did not get the same feelings from food that I get now. I also did not experience the same energy after eating as I do now—I now eat more sodium, sugar, and refined carbohydrate based on my intuitive desires for them. But according to the HEI, this is less healthy than the bland diet of deficiency I was on years prior.

Your intuitive experience of eating can fill in a lot of the gaps from the various nutritional ideologies you may be fascinated with, whether it be keto, paleo, or a "plant-based" lifestyle (eating cow meat is plant based as ruminant animals like cows recycle plants), and you can use it to understand how not just food, but even the events surrounding eating food (cooking, your mood, social life, watching TV, etc.) affect your health.

One more reason I must bring forth on why the HEI is incomplete is that there is absolutely no mention of *spices* in it. Since *billions* of people, from all of Asia, South America, Central America, Mexico, and Africa eat spices almost daily, and up to several times per day with meals, the HEI fails to factor in a central component of eating. The nutrients in foods aren't all that determine health. The way foods are mixed, flavored, prepared, and enjoyed with company all help create a satisfying and nourishing experience that is far too abstract for nutrition science to attempt to study.

Although the HEI is a useful tool for research purposes, it clearly demonstrates to me how fragmented our thinking is with our food. We separate it into categories and think that eating enough categories is ideal for our health. According to the HEI a balanced diet includes some milk, but not everyone does well with cow's milk. According to the HEI we should limit our cholesterol intake to below 300 milligrams a day, less than the amount in two eggs. According to the HEI, more fruits and vegetables are better for our health. What about the seasonal availability of these foods? What about traditional diets that don't include a lot of fruits but produce robust health, fewer cavities, and better bone structure as discovered by Weston A. Price (a dentist who traveled the world to study indigenous populations and tooth health, in the 1920s and discovered that traditional diets were far better).

Along with the equally incomplete dietary recommendations the U.S. government has given to its citizens for decades, the HEI is a microcosm and epitome of the way we discuss health—a perfect explanation for why we are so confused. There's a lot missing from the HEI, and I believe we can fill in the gaps by learning to follow our bodies and operate more from feel rather than by drawing broad conclusions from population-based studies.

The discussion on what a truly healthy diet is simply beyond the focus of this book, but my beliefs certainly are influenced by Weston A. Price in part, as it's fascinating that there seems to be a relationship between nutrient-dense foods in the diet, namely animal foods, and better bone structure as well as physical beauty,[10] which is a subject expounded upon in Deep Nutrition, by Dr. Catherine Shanahan.[11] However, since we continue to evolve, suggesting that we should follow the exact diet of our evolutionary past may be incomplete as well.

Saturated Fat

In the summer of 2017, the American Heart Association published a scientific report on saturated fat and cardiovascular disease (CVD).[12] They made it sound quite fancy by calling it a "Presidential Advisory." The purpose of this report was to summarize the research on the role of saturated fat in promoting cardiovascular disease, to I suppose update practitioners, as well as the public on why they should take statin drugs. They picked four "core" trials—all several decades old— to support their hypothesis. One section of the report created a stir in the health blogosphere. They singled out coconut oil and said that they could not recommend its consumption based on its high saturated fat content.

> ...because coconut oil increases LDL cholesterol, a cause of CVD, and has no known offsetting favorable effects, we advise against the use of coconut oil.

In that report, studies from the 1960s that examined saturated fat (SFA—the A is for acid) versus polyunsaturated fat (PUFA, for polyunsaturated fatty acids) formed the basis for the authors' conclusions that saturated fat consumption should be limited. In those remarkably old trials, replacing SFAs with PUFAs seemed to reduce the number of heart attacks.

But they purposely ignored another study, the Minnesota Coronary Experiment (MCE), which took place from 1968-1973, and contradicted two decades of prior research on the subject.[13] Consequently, results from the MCE weren't published until over a decade after the experiment was finished—a classic case of publication bias. In the MCE, one group of participants consumed a diet richer in PUFAs, and the other, a diet richer in SFAs, just as in all the prior studies.

Cholesterol levels declined predictably in the group consuming more PUFAs, enhancing their image as usual—at least in the eyes of those who have fallen for the lipid hypothesis, which purports that saturated fat and cholesterol intake increases the risk of heart disease (see my article summarizing the research on dietary cholesterol and cardiovascular disease risk[14]). Unexpectedly however, cardiovascular disease incidence and mortality increased quite significantly in this group. The findings of the study were published in the *British Medical Journal*:

> Findings from the Minnesota Coronary Experiment add to growing evidence that incomplete publication has contributed to overestimation of the benefits of replacing saturated fat with vegetable oils rich in linoleic acid.

Linoleic acid by the way, is one of the major PUFAs found in food. The AHA explained why they didn't include this study in their core trials: the MCE included too many trans fats in the experimental diets. I decided to head to a local medical library to investigate these "core" trials myself. I knew that margarine was a popular food back in those times, so I wondered if it was included in the diets within these studies. I requested articles from the closed stacks of this library and began reading one of the four trials, the Finnish Mental Hospital Study (FMHS).[15]

In the FMHS, participants comprised patients at two mental hospitals. At each hospital, patients started on one diet for six years, then switched to another diet for six more years. This type of design is called a cross-over design. One diet was a control diet with over 50-60% of fats coming from the saturated type (the NORM diet), and the other was a "serum cholesterol-lowering" diet (the SCL diet), with 35-45% of fats coming from the polyunsaturated variety.

The researchers measured serum cholesterol levels and examined deaths and incidence of cardiovascular disease (CVD) before and after the study. They measured CVD incidence directly, by counting deaths, and indirectly, with electrocardiography, a technique that charts the electrical activity of different parts of the heart.

This study listed the foods consumed in each diet and at each hospital, unlike the other three studies in the "core" group, which I also obtained in the closed stacks. In both the NORM and SCL diets, the total amount of fat was kept the same, but the ratio of saturated to polyunsaturated fats differed. The NORM diet had a higher ratio of saturated fat to polyunsaturated fat than the SCL diet. In the diet designed to lower cholesterol (SCL), butter was replaced with "soft" margarine. In the other diet (NORM), increased concentrations of saturated fat were achieved by increasing the amount of milk and butter fats, as well as "common" margarine.

I had no idea what the difference was between these types of margarine, but one *New York Times* article from 1984 seems to highlight the difference.[16]

> Overall, tub margarines have the best ratios, often 2 to 1 and even 2.5 to 1 of polyunsaturated to saturated fat. The reason is that they contain less hydrogenated oil than many stick margarines; hydrogenation, the process of hardening oil, turns some of the unsaturated fat to saturated.

Fatty acids contain two components: a carbon chain of variable length, and a carboxylic acid group. In the chain, each carbon atom holds hands with an adjacent carbon atom—this is called a bond. Each bond represents the sharing of two electrons. Thus, a single bond represents the sharing of two electrons, a double bond: four; and a triple bond: six.

Think of each carbon as having four arms, arranged like a compass: north, south, east, and west (although that's not what it looks like in three-dimensional space). In a saturated fatty acid, each carbon in the carbon chain is holding hands with two other carbon atoms, and two hydrogen atoms. This fulfills its need to have eight electrons around it. In this arrangement, there are no more electrons to share, and no space for additional atoms to bond with. It is saturated.

In an unsaturated fatty acid, we find carbons in the chain forming double bonds with adjacent carbons. Thus, one carbon in the chain might have a single bond with one carbon, a double bond with the other adjacent carbon, and a single bond with a hydrogen, to maintain eight electrons in its outer valence shell.

A *monounsaturated* fatty acid contains just one double bond in its chain. A polyunsaturated fatty acid has *multiple* double bonds in its chain. These two kinds of fatty acids are the ones that can become hydrogenated; a hydrogen can attack the double bonds, facilitating a transfer of electrons, turning them into single bonds by bonding to the carbon itself. The once poly- or monounsaturated fatty acid becomes saturated if all the double bonds in its chain get attacked by hydrogens.

This is exactly what happens when a vegetable oil rich in PUFAs is heated to high temperatures for a prolonged period of time, as in frying: some of the double bonds become hydrogenated, and it is now classifiable as a partially hydrogenated fatty acid. In addition to an increased number of hydrogenated fatty acids, some of the existing polyunsaturated fatty acids in the vegetable oil change their configuration from a cis- to a trans- formation during the hydrogenation process. This formation has to do with the "kinks," or bends in the chain as a result of double bonding. The trans-fatty acids resulting from hydrogenation have a configuration that is not found in nature, and thus, they aren't classified as polyunsaturated fatty acids.

PUFAs stay liquid at room temperature, whereas saturated fats, abundant in butter, ghee, coconut oil, and lard, are solid at room temperature. Tub margarines, which contain more polyunsaturated fats, were the "soft" margarine used in the Finnish Mental Hospital Study, and the stick margarine is the "common" one, which is harder and contains more saturated fatty acids (from the hydrogenation process).

In the FMHS, common margarine (the one with more trans-fat) was incorporated into the control diet (NORM diet) to keep the percentage of SFA among the rest of the fats at 50-60%. The SCL diet contained more soft margarine, and thus fewer trans-fats. In this study, those on the SCL diet saw slightly fewer deaths from CVD, as well as fewer abnormal ECG changes. This supported the the AHA's hypothesis, or rather, preconceived notion which they would never think twice about defending.

Unsurprisingly, when results don't support the AHA's hypothesis, like in the Minnesota Coronary Experiment which had far stronger results, the AHA chose to ignore them. There was no mention in their Presidential Advisory about the daily consumption of trans-fats in the Finnish Mental Hospital Study. Thus, the AHA is hypocritical, among other pejoratives.

WHEN WE READ ABOUT the latest research from a press release, only the headline gets through to us. We get the "main point." Few media outlets ever cite the original source of the study (since they're focused on ad revenue there isn't much incentive for them to share a link to the original source because you'd end up leaving their website) and few people are curious enough to critically read the study. Even fewer people have the knowledge on how to read these studies, what to look for, and how to interpret the findings. This creates mass confusion.

And this is why Medium published a piece[17] on this issue titled "Is the American Heart Association a terrorist organization?" Their point was that the AHA was spreading propaganda, not facts, which could harm millions of people. The authors of the presidential advisory are certainly highly educated and have the credentials that we hold with high regard in society, but they also know that most people have no idea how to interpret research, and perhaps they take advantage of this from time to time to support their agenda. Their confirmation biases are too obvious.

Days after this report was published, Mazola, a vegetable oil manufacturing company shared a picture on their Facebook that read "swapping coconut oil with corn oil may reduce the risk of heart disease by about 30%." This was most likely not a coincidence. And there's no data to support this fact. The core studies in the AHA's report did not compare coconut oil to corn oil, and this thinking is a great example of the pervasiveness of reductionism in the marketing tactics of various organizations, along with corporate bias and bad science.

Hold on—it gets worse. A very important point in the Finnish Mental Hospital Study that the AHA also left out of their report was drug use between groups. The participants in this study were on psychiatric medications that affect the heart, including phenothiazine antipsychotics, such as thoridazine, and tricyclic antidepressants such as imipramine and amitriptyline. A plethora of articles from the '60s expressed concern that phenothiazines may have been causing sudden unexplained deaths,[18,19,20] precipitated by a malfunctioning of the heart.

One of the abnormal ECG changes the researchers looked for in the FMHS was pathologic Q waves. They claimed that the drugs the participants were on were not likely to cause any abnormal changes to the Q wave. I performed a quick search and found a study performed in South Africa which found significant prolongation of the QTc interval in about a quarter of the subjects taking the medication.[21] In the '60s, again, it was already well-known that this drug produced abnormal and concerning changes to the ECG.[22]

And what about those tricyclic antidepressants? Well, they're also associated with abnormal changes to the ECG and sudden unexplained death.[23] Participants on the NORM diet in one of the two hospitals took *twice as many* TCAs than when they were on the SCL diet (recall that this was a crossover design, so participants spent six years on one diet then switched to the other). This group also saw the most deaths and ECG changes, although the total amount of deaths was pretty small. The authors of the FMHS didn't think much of this, as they suggested that the drugs the participants were on weren't known to cause any of the ECG changes they were looking for.

I would expect so called "experts," "professionals," and "scientists" at the American Heart Association who wrote the presidential advisory to acknowledge these facts, but there is no mention of it in their report. Instead, saturated fat was the sole villain. Not drugs that cause sudden unexplained death (which in most cases involve a malfunctioning of the heart and are thus grouped into cardiovascular mortality) or trans-fats. I'm going to have to agree with Medium. The

AHA is akin to a terrorist organization, spreading lies and propaganda for personal gain in lieu of the greater good.

Considering the daily dose of margarine and cardiotoxic drugs in the FMHS, it seems quite silly to blame saturated fat on cardiovascular disease, and then even more silly to blame red meat or coconut oil as a cause of CVD. The most abundant fatty acid in steak is not a saturated fatty acid; it's oleic acid, the same monounsaturated fat in olive oil.[24] Yet most people think of red meat as a prime source of "unhealthy" fats. Again, misinterpreted, biased, and not-even-properly-read science.

Why are some people still interested in framing saturated fat, just one constituent among many of some of the foods we eat, as a bad thing for our health? Why is it that we can go back and forth in citing studies that implicate saturated fat in CVD and others that find no association whatsoever? Quite simply because there are some powerful organizations that can benefit financially from this information being disseminated to the public. I think you can figure out who those are. Sugar companies, vegetable oil companies, and of course, the AHA, which benefits from the notion that lowering cholesterol is better for our health, thus making statins an attractive option for the treatment and prevention of cardiovascular disease.

The studies in the 1960s that replaced SFAs with PUFAs were interested in showing that the reduction in total cholesterol levels in the PUFA group mediated the relationship between PUFAs and reduced cardiovascular disease incidence. When they found out that in the MCE the trend was reversed, they ignored it, just like they ignore studies that question the cholesterol hypothesis. The AHA can only be expected to continue to maintain the assertion that reducing cholesterol is a good preventive strategy for cardiovascular disease.

The story behind the AHA's report, and the story behind the studies cited in that report, paint a convoluted picture. The AHA isn't the only organization influencing health policy that bathes in murky waters. I used to think that I should examine things on a case-by-case basis, but I feel now that based on the source, we can predict what will be said. Information is biased, but thankfully, in many cases we can clearly see where the bias comes from as we'll discuss next.

Explicit Bias

Once I understood where the bias came from, I almost felt relieved. It's comforting to know that we can at least understand how policy and advice can get mixed up with the motives of wealthy, power-hungry corporations. Below are three examples where my trust in nutrition science fell into a dark abyss.

1. Tufts University and Kellogg's® Froot Loops®

In 2009, the dean of the Freidman School of Nutrition Science and Food Policy at Tufts University, Eileen T. Kennedy, proclaimed Froot Loops® was a healthy breakfast choice based on government dietary guidelines. She was the president of the Smart Choices program, an industry-backed effort to promote shitty foods.

Foods that met the criteria for this program were labeled with a green check mark. Well, I should rephrase. The packaging that the food-like product came in was labeled with a green check mark. The companies involved in the Smart Choices program included Coca-cola, Pepsico, Kraft Foods, Kellogg, Walmart, ConAgra, the National Dairy Council, Wrigley, and others.[25] Other sponsors included The American Diabetic Association, the American Dietetic Association, and the Heart and Stroke Foundation (Canada's version of the AHA).

Behind the whole effort was the American Society of Nutrition, which publishes much of the nutrition research in the United States.

They have four journals, two of which are in the top 10 nutrition journals worldwide: the *American Clinical Journal of Nutrition* and the *Journal of Nutrition*. They're peer-reviewed, and supposed to be of high quality. But considering the ties between industry and research, it's hard for me to imagine that the American Society of Nutrition has any interest in our health, just like the AHA.

2. Organic Apples Suck

The same year, I entered the University of Maryland to study nutrition. I had a small scholarship and was excited to study what I was passionate about. In my first semester, I took a class called "Introduction to Nutrition and Food Science," which was taught by the dean of the Nutrition and Food Science Program, a very funny Asian guy who was seen smiling most of the time.

One day in class he held up two apples. "Look at this apple, it's bright, red, and shiny! And look at this one. It's dull, small, and has a hole in it. Well this one's organic (pointing to the duller apple), and this brighter bigger one is not!" His charisma made it hard for the class not to laugh, but my head turned hot. I was about to storm out of the classroom, as I saw at that moment I was in the wrong place. I was 18, impulsive, idealistic, ignorant, and ready to change the world.

Shortly thereafter in a discussion section for the class, we discussed a variety of food topics. One of them was raw milk. The teaching assistant (TA) for the section played a YouTube video of a farmer explaining the health benefits of raw milk. To an audience of college students, her speech sounded quite woo-woo. It wasn't scientific. And thus, it wasn't acceptable. Everyone laughed at her for the claims she made, including the TA. I stood there, perplexed. Why didn't we at least try to listen to what she was saying? What if there was some merit to it after all? I changed my major next semester. If I was more intuitive though, I would have just dropped out.

3. Registered Dietitians (RDs)

Most RDs who decide to follow me on Instagram seem to have escaped the brainwashing in most nutrition and dietetics programs. But one recent follower didn't. She recommends Belvita breakfast biscuits, a Nabisco product, on her page. My father shipped me a package of them once as a gift, but I gave them away to a homeless person, because it is yet another product of food corporations and isn't real food. My intuition doesn't recognize it. It doesn't want it. (You could argue that this perception comes from a strong bias I have, and sure, that's a fair argument, but you haven't gotten to part III yet, so hold on tight).

This RD says however that these biscuits contain 4g of fiber, and 4g of protein. Well, my Ikea table that I've left outside in the rain that is somehow still standing has plenty of fiber and proteins too. Logically, it's a great reason to eat food. But intuitively, it's not.

Fiber, protein, and other nutrients that make a food sound good logically are marketing tools. Having a certain amount of these nutrients can qualify the food to meet some standard for being healthy, or become "AHA approved", with a shiny red check mark. None of this is about health. And this RD's Instagram page is simply an advertisement for various food-products created by companies that influenced her education.

Qualitative Data vs. Quantitative Data

Apart from bias and misinterpretation, there is another very important reason why we shouldn't just rely on nutrition science to determine what to eat: quantitative data informs us differently than qualitative data does. Quantitative data is the basis for the biological sciences. Qualitative data is used in the social sciences. Epidemiology is one quantitative approach that holds promise in finding trends between health behaviors and health outcomes (a commonly studied outcome is the incidence of a specific disease for example). But when it comes to nutrition, its results can be quite difficult to draw any conclusions from.

The grandfather of epidemiology, at least according to the Western science taught in our academic institutions, is John Snow. His passion project was cholera, which killed tens-of-thousands of people in London in the mid-1800s. The widely-accepted theory at the time, and the one promoted by the Registrar of London, General William Farr, was the miasmatic theory of disease. Farr believed that the disease was transmitted by a cloud hovering over the population at the lowest altitudes. Those living at lower altitudes were thus more likely to contract the illness.

Snow disagreed; his observations contradicted the mainstream theory. He found that there were two water supplies in the city, both of which came from the Thames river. Sewage systems back in those days were not well-developed, and thus waste was regularly dumped into the river or into cesspools adjacent to it.[26] One of the water companies, the Lambeth Company, obtained water near a highly contaminated part of the river: a literal shit-hole. Snow hypothesized that people who drank this water were more likely to get cholera than those drinking water from the other company, Southwark and Vauxhall Co. I hope I would have guessed the same thing.

He went house-to-house, tabulating deaths from cholera with water source. The results were strikingly obvious. Those who obtained water from the company that operated near the shithole were far more likely to get cholera. His findings were so promising, they persuaded the adamant William Farr to look further into the issue. Snow's ideas however were still not accepted for some time, and after many more preventable deaths.

Snow proved that cholera was transmitted in the water. After people drank contaminated water, they often died shortly thereafter. Those who drank uncontaminated water did not die from cholera at such a high rate. Snow's ideas weren't accepted initially, but his methods paved the path for modern day epidemiology. Epidemiology is very useful in tracking the spread of dangerous pathogens like cholera that have a clear cause-and-effect relationship between transmission and illness. When it comes to nutrition however, associations aren't as clear.

Coffee for example has been a controversial drink for diabetics, as it can raise blood sugar. Meta-analyses however have found a negative relationship between coffee consumption and diabetes risk;[27] this means that the more coffee people drink, the less their chance of developing diabetes. But the effect of coffee and diabetes risk is very different than the effect of cholera on life. The effects of these two things have a very different time course. And as you may guess, coffee is simply far weaker than cholera.

Although it is fairly clear from the robust meta-analyses and systematic reviews on the subject that coffee does not cause diabetes, under the right circumstance, it might still have the possibility. A high carbohydrate meal with caffeinated coffee for example temporarily lowered insulin sensitivity in one study with healthy young male participants after a carbohydrate meal.[28] Studies like that however examine short term associations. One drink caused a temporary decline in insulin sensitivity. This doesn't mean those men are at an increased risk of diabetes. But it begs the question, is it the coffee consumption preventing diabetes or the activities people who drink coffee partake in that prevents diabetes? We often won't know the answer to this chicken-or-egg question when browsing nutrition epidemiology.

Food is powerful, but not as powerful alone, as we eat them with other foods and over long periods of time. A single food simply isn't as potent as a drug or a pathogenic organism. Epidemiology may not aid us in determining if foods are healthy or unhealthy for us very easily because it's hard to tease out one food in the context of our whole diet. Statistician John Ionnidis even calls nutritional epidemiology a "utopian endeavor," as the benefit from any healthy-sounding thing seen in most studies is so small, the overall finding just isn't all that likely to be true. I've felt the same way for seven years.

Although the HEI is based on epidemiological data that has found higher fruit and vegetable intakes to be associated with lower all-cause and cardiovascular mortality, does that mean we should all be eating more fruits and vegetables if we don't naturally crave them? If we don't crave fruits and vegetables, maybe it means we don't want them, and don't need them. Maybe we need more meat, a food that is also highly nutritious, but which authorities suggest limiting, due to irrational fears of saturated fat and cholesterol.

The "what if I'm not craving it" question is one I began pondering after realizing that my own diet was constructed quite logically and off seemingly sound nutrition science that still conflicted with my appetite's desires. I was starting to be pulled more and more by my intuition. And once I began following it, I felt *better*.

Although we all have many similarities, we have differences that influence what foods we thrive on. Epidemiological data cannot inform us about these individual needs however, as the premise for those studies is that we're all the same. The strength in those studies comes from having a large sample size of *homogenous* individuals. Being homogenous ensures a greater chance of capturing a true effect of whatever is being investigated, whether it be coffee for diabetes, or saturated fat for cardiovascular disease. If everyone in those studies was different, it would be difficult to draw out cause and effect. That's why larger sample sizes increase the statistical power of these studies.

Quantitative data can also be manipulated to favor one point of view over another. The statistics performed after the completion of the experiment can be reported in a way to make some things look better than others. This type of bias isn't uncommon in science.

Quantitative data also communicates information in a different language than qualitative data; this language can be confusing and intimidating to the layman. The numbers attached to our health attempt to paint a picture of what's going on inside. But they can't fully explain the experience. Two people may have similar numbers but completely different experiences.

So instead of relying on quantitative data, we are going to use *qualitative* data. We are going to discard every single quantitative aspect of food, including carbs, fats, and proteins, there is, and start from scratch. We will think of the *qualities* of fats, proteins, and carbohydrates instead, but we will not think about them in terms of weight, carbon-chain length, or molecular structure (quantitative data). I know that quantitative thinking can be quite interesting. It's like doing a puzzle. For others it's just a headache.

Qualitative data is abstract and can be just as confusing as quantitative data. But the benefit for you is that you deal with it every day. You receive qualitative data from the foods you eat *every single day*. So don't you find it crazy that when we discuss health, we don't have guidelines on what this qualitative data means? We don't' talk about how we feel when we eat.

We talk just about vitamins, minerals, and other measurable things in our food. Modern medicine is mostly quantitative as well, and this can lead to viewing the body as a series of numbers, treating those numbers, and ignoring the qualitative aspects of the patient. Homeopathy in contrast is mostly qualitative, and is completely ostracized by the medical community. It's in a completely different language, and exists within a different paradigm: the paradigm of the holographic universe, which we'll get to in chapter 3.

What is qualitative data anyway? Qualitative data include feelings and sensations. Many parts of the physical exam a doctor may perform include a mix of qualitative and quantitative data. For example, a thyroid gland may feel swollen. Since this is approximated with physical touch, there is no grading system. It might feel boggy too, or firm. Maybe it's difficult to palpate. All of that is qualitative information.

Depression is another illness that is mostly qualitative. However, in order for doctors to diagnose it and understand it, the data is transformed via surveys and inventories. Patients take a survey and get a score. This score is a quantitative measure of their illness that is easier for the practitioner to diagnose and interpret.

Qualitative data on the other hand is what you will be gathering about food and your appetite and anything surrounding it influencing your eating habits in your intuitive eating journey. It's important to stay in this realm, as one of the most potent intuition-blocking factors we'll discuss in chapter 5 is logic. So if you're a compulsive note-taker or tracker, you will need to let go of your urge to make lists about all the qualitative data you are about to accumulate from connecting to your food. The experience must be internalized for you to learn. But of course, there will be exercises where you are required to write stuff down. It's just important to realize that connecting to the sensations and experiences may be hampered if we constantly try to write everything down.

So Why Doesn't Mainstream Nutrition Advice Rely on Qualitative Data?

There are a couple important reasons why in nutrition science, and in Western culture, qualitative data isn't valued enough. One is that research supports academic institutions and corporations. Professors need to establish themselves by conducting good research to keep their jobs. Research needs to be performed to better understand what's working and what isn't. Better diagnostic techniques can be developed. Better procedures can be developed. New technologies can be put to the test. We need research. It's just unfortunate that traditional systems of medicine are viewed as inferior because they have not been translated to properly to fit within the Western scientific paradigm.

So capitalism is one reason, and there are pros and cons to this. But apart from capitalism, another reason why mainstream nutrition advice is lacking in qualitative and intuitive data is due to a lack of culture within our own culture. In America, most of us aren't originally from America. My parents are from India, but I'm not very Indian in terms of my culture, religious beliefs, and eating habits. I love Indian food, but I don't yet cook as well as people in India do. They grow up cooking, learning about spices, and connecting to food. We live in a consumer culture where this interaction with food is often derailed by the interests of corporations, which include serving us highly palatable foods which aren't good for us. That's why we're fat and rank very low in terms of overall health.

Imagine if people from rural areas of Turkey were presented with American food: burgers, chips, fries, and Kool-Aid for example. I'd expect half of these willing participants to vomit. These people from Turkey know what good food looks and tastes like. Americans who don't know food well, due to an absence of connection with food in our culture, may be more prone to eating widely available, inexpensive, and nutritionally devoid junk foods. If we grew up learning how to make delicious food with healthy and natural ingredients instead of artificial ones, would we be as prone to become addicted to malnourishing but calorie-dense foods? I'd think not, but it's possible.

What's the solution? The solution isn't to find a cultural paradigm and adopt its set of dietary beliefs. One solution however is to first learn the difference between food-like products, which often carry deceptive advertising claims, from real food, and then stop labeling it as much. More succinctly, this means educate and then intuit. If we only intuited, we would take much longer to figure out what foods are best for us.

For the average American, learning about the types of foods on the market is very important. This person does not know how food is labeled and may think that unhealthy food items are good for them when they might not be that great. On the other hand, the health-conscious consumer who has developed stronger beliefs about what foods are healthy and has a basic understanding of the chemistry within foods will benefit from learning to enjoy food more and labeling it less. Wherever you are in your understanding, you can use the exercises and ideas coming up to help you make more intuitive choices, which in theory, are better choices.

This process involves a lot of trial and error, and it may result in greater appreciation of food. Perhaps you'll experiment with foods from different cultures and be able to construct a unique diet for yourself that combines the elements of each culture's cuisine that works for you. Or if you're more into science rather than traditional methods of eating, you can use the ideas in this book to better understand how much protein, fat, and carbs you need in your diet, without even measuring them!

You may find, like I did, that you need starchy carbs sometimes to feel your best. Without them, your strength, muscle mass, and energy levels decline, despite the cosmetic benefit of being slightly leaner. You can then determine when you need to eat them, based on symptoms and signs you've been paying greater attention to as a result of the exercises in this book and simply by increasing your self-awareness.

These types of subjective and qualitative pieces of information aren't valued enough in nutrition discussions. For me personally, it's the most valuable because it relates the most directly to quality of life. When you eat the right foods for your body and at the right time, based on your activity levels and day-to-day needs, you will be able to do more of what you want to and need to with your life.

There are a multitude of other reasons why most nutrition advice is not qualitative or intuitive, and they will be discussed more in chapter 5. One very important reason discussed there is logical thinking, which goes hand-in-hand with the quantitative nature of nutrition science. Science relies on the logical mind. This mind finds patterns, conducts experiments, and gets to the root cause of the problem. Its emphasis in problem-solving can often suppress intuition.

Intuition is always with us, but when we train ourselves to emphasize logic over intuition, it won't be able to work as effectively. It's a simple case of use it or lose it. It's like our feet. Feet contain muscles, tendons, and ligaments. We don't use them as much when we wear shoes. We still have those feet, but we don't engage them to their fullest by always covering them up with shoes. Similarly, when logic predominates, intuition takes a back seat. So all we have to do it honor it and take the shoes off from time to time.

Taking Intuition with Us

How did TCM doctors figure out, as well as every medicine man or woman, shaman, healer, and grandmother on the planet, that ginger helped fight colds and the flu? They evaluated the qualitative aspects of ginger, rather than its chemical constituents (which weren't known anyway). Metaphorically, it's the energy of ginger that revealed its uses. In this case, when I say energy, I don't mean kilojoules; I mean the soul, the heart, and essence of something.

The following account is a description of ginger's energy from "Between Heaven and Earth: A Guide to Chinese Medicine" by Harriet Beinfield and Efrem Korngold.[29]

> Ginger, familiar to us all, illustrates how configuration, color, taste, odor, and nature correlate with use. Ginger is yellow, fragrant, and sweet, which corresponds to Earth (Stomach and Spleen), and pungent and spicy, which corresponds to Metal (Lung and Large Intestine). It has a warm nature and juicy texture, so it warms and moisturizes, making it suitable for Cold and Dryness-based digestive and respiratory conditions (such as a flu with thirst, dry cough, chills, and diarrhea). The spiciness of raw ginger decongests Qi (relieving symptoms such as cramps, nausea, and indigestion, including motion and morning sickness) and dispels Wind and phlegm (relieving symptoms such as fever, cough, and dizziness). When roasted, it has a greater warming and drying action, eliminating Cold and Dampness from the body's core (relieving symptoms like chilliness, water retention, and poor circulation).

Ginger's qualities include pungency, spiciness, juiciness, yellowness, fragrance, and sweetness. Raw ginger has different qualities than cooked ginger and thus different medicinal applications. Not only does ginger have different qualities so do different conditions and people. Ginger is good for a lot of conditions, but not all, because of its qualities according to TCM. Of course, these qualities will sound like mumbo-jumbo to people who are accustomed to studying cell biology, pharmacology, and other quantitative disciplines.

But despite the lack of modern biological sciences thousands of years ago, I believe that a balanced meal according to TCM is far tastier than the balanced meals recommended by the United States Department of Agriculture with their MyPlate concept. MyPlate recommends portions of meat, vegetables, fruit, grains, and dairy products. The idea is that a balanced meal contains calculated portions of these foods. This idea is commonly applied to food-like products designed to be healthy.

Chinese cuisine in contrast emphasizes the balance of qualities in a meal. Contrast a meal consisting of brothy soup, herbs, lime, noodles, and thinly sliced meat with Soylent. Which one sounds better to you? Oh, Soylent...really? You must be a *cough* sociopath.

It's not just China of course that knows what a balanced diet is. Any traditional society of our past as well as present understands this concept. As humans we have been far more connected to nature in the past than now, and the ramifications of this concept on what we eat I believe could completely change what we view is healthy and not healthy. Out of all the ideas that I've been exposed to, the idea of eating "naturally" has stuck with me. But my initial interpretation of what was "natural" was far from it, as I only concerned myself with the foods I consumed.

Now, my interpretation is of eating "naturally" has everything to do with the mindset. I believe the "natural" mindset required to eat naturally is a mindset traditional cultures have. It's a mindset that requires us to be highly intuitive and connected with nature. It's not a mindset that scrutinizes food labels and freaks out about ingredients which aren't "natural." It's a mindset that understands when to eat, how to eat, and what good food really tastes like. It's not a mindset that people in the fitness industry promote. It's not a mindset that most underweight models have with their food. But it's a mindset that can create peace, calm, and a healthy relationship with food, and of course, excellent health. And certainly, it's a mindset that cares about quality food.

And that's why when I was drinking kale juice to be healthy, I was far less "natural" than I am now when I drink coffee with milk and sugar. When I drank kale juice, I operated from logos. When I add cream and sugar to my coffee, I operate from *pathos* (emotion). In fact, I don't even think about it. All I know is that I want some sweet and I want my drink to be a bit more concentrated. But when I drink pour overs, it's a different story. I can drink that black because it has more flavor and often the sugar and cream ruin it for me.

If you crave pancakes let's say, maybe that means you need a significant portion of carbohydrates. Isn't this how we ate in our evolutionary past? How did we alienate ourselves from our instincts so much that we only consider the food's quantitative properties as a contributor to its health benefits? Our own unique needs play a large role in a food's benefits, and we will discuss this at length in future chapters.

I think the most important thing we can learn from our wise ancestors about eating healthfully has nothing to do with food itself. It's their *connection* with nature that we can learn from. This connection is what informed them what to eat. When we analyze data on our computers and read nutrition science, we don't connect to nature in the same way. When we're actually in nature, we start to connect with it, understand it, and *feel* it. As a result, we eat intuitively. And that's how we're meant to eat.

Why Intuition Matters

Your intuition is a simple thing. It just wants some attention here and there, and doesn't ask for too much. We used it not just to decide what to eat, but who to mate with, who to let in our tribe, and for many other reasons related to survival in our evolutionary past. We still have it of course; it's not going away. But many forces derail our intuition, negatively affecting our relationship with food and the health benefits from it that we seek. It's counterintuitive that logical approaches to eating could be worse for our health than not thinking about food as much at all.

And that's why intuitive eating is more important than ever today. It adds subjectivity and personalization to the health equation. In contrast, science aims to be objective and assumes that subjects in any group are all the same: homogenous, as discussed earlier. But we're not all the same. It's why not everyone who takes vitamin D sees their vitamin D levels go up,[30] or why not everyone who starts exercising sees an increase in their maximum oxygen carrying capacity. [31] Researchers are well aware of this, but homogeneity is assumed in studies because it's easier to determine cause and effect this way. Cause and effect cannot be determined as easily when we take a whole food, combine it with many other variables, factor in individual variability, *and* observe how it's affecting people's health.

Because of these inherent problems research has to deal with, the results of scientific experiments cannot provide more than an *estimate*. Whether we're talking about how many cigarettes you need to smoke before you get lung cancer or how many calories you need to burn before you achieve a six-pack, the science cannot ever give you an exact answer. It was never really meant to, but somehow, we decided it should. Some genius came up with the idea that there are 3500 calories in one pound of fat, and consequently misled people for decades.

When you use attempt to intuit what foods are working for you and what aren't, you will be the scientist in charge of your experiments. If you have a condition like Hashimoto's for instance, figuring out what foods work for you and what doesn't will require self-study and lots of trial and error. If you are free from health conditions, you can focus on things like your mood, energy, and digestion, all of which will be discussed in Chapter 6.

Although intuition is abstract and imprecise, we can use it to **fact-check** the results of a study. Say a study comes out that says the ketogenic diet relieves symptoms of Hashimoto's and lowers antibody count. You go on the diet, hoping for symptom relief, but don't experience an improvement. Should you stick to it because the study found that it might work? Maybe not. Unfortunately, this is how many people approach health. They stick to something that isn't working because they heard it might work, but aren't listening to their body telling them right then and there that it's not working. As anathema as anecdotal evidence is to the scientific community, I think we can learn a lot from it when it's done right.

Anecdotes that involve fiction aren't helpful. But when we carefully observe our symptoms and aim to correlate them with what we ate and with other factors in our lifestyle, we can make important discoveries about our health. This process is essential for the intuitive eater. There's no guide that you can blindly follow. You have to be aware of your body. With time, it takes very little effort and feels natural.

Once you get the hang of it, you'll figure out when you're hungry and when you're full. You'll then fact check this by repeating it over and over again. You'll remember the feeling of fullness and will rely on this memory for future reference. In contrast, if this book was about scientific techniques, we'd measure ghrelin, a hormone that is released when we're hungry. And that could be a fun obsession. We could correlate ghrelin levels with perceived hunger and fullness, but that would cause more of a headache than I'm already giving you most likely and may not be as accurate as we'd expect.

The Battle of Listening to My Damn Intuition

One of my favorite teachers, Mr. B, taught my 7th grade history class. He was a bald male in his 30s who happily told us that he had a crush on one of our other teachers, as well as Jennifer Lopez. One day he asked us a standard question about something we recently learned. An answer came to me fairly immediately, but I wasn't sure if it was correct. I decided against raising my hand to answer the question. No one raised their hand in fact. After a short anticipatory silence, he told us the answer. I was right. Damn it! I missed out on some easy validation.

What I didn't do was listen to my intuition. Now, the answer that popped into my head may have not been from intuitive insight; it may have been from what we think of as memory. But of course, memory and intuition overlap, depending on which theories you subscribe to. That is beyond our scope here, but McTaggart argues that our memories are stored in a quantum field, rather than somewhere in the brain as is typically thought of (this thought will be expounded upon in the next chapter).

Regardless of the mechanism, there is one peculiar similarity between just about every answer that has ever came into my head in class prompted by a teacher's question that I also was too afraid to blurt out: the answer was a bit hazy. It wasn't an immediate "aha." It wasn't something I looked over the day before. It was something more distant my consciousness was trying to access.

These nuances are important. I don't want to pretend that every idea that comes into our head comes from intuition, the definition of which is abstract and not entirely proven to be true. However, my definition, and the definition others have come up with, have considerable overlap, indicating a high amount of validity.

Perhaps I was also just very shy in class. As I grew older and became more confident, I blurted out more answers. But the answers that I blurted out were often wrong, and felt different to me than those correct answers that were on the tip of my tongue, but that I didn't feel confident enough to blurt out. I do believe the latter scenario is mediated by intuition, because intuition is always right. It's also sometimes a bit fuzzy, unfortunately.

Eventually, I did blurt out more correct answers. My goal was to stop ignoring those intuitive answers, and this was the battle. The battle was between my logical mind, the mind that has been trained in schools for two decades, and a growing intuitive mind that prospers when I remember to turn the logical mind off.

Since that day in 7th grade, I've made it a goal to follow my gut instincts. It's been nearly fifteen years since that day, and all I can say is I'm beginning to connect with intuition more than ever, and it's difficult to explain to those who haven't experienced it. That's why I think this book will connect most to those who are already on their way to becoming more intuitive. If I read this book with the mind and the lens with which I viewed the world five years ago, it wouldn't make much sense to me, even though I wanted to become more intuitive. I just wasn't there yet.

Those who have experienced the benefits of following intuitive insight will resonate with the message here, and those who haven't may find it strange and confusing, although I hope they'd be open. It's conventionally thought that intuitive moments, such as where you and your friend are texting each other at the same exact time out of the blue, are just coincidences. But what if they're more than that?

My intuition was suppressed throughout my whole life; I was raised by immigrant parents who emphasized education over everything else. This upbringing caused me to value science, logic, and reasoning ability, which I believe was a major reason why I experimented with so many diets that were metabolism-suppressing, while tunneling deep into the rabbit holes of logic supporting each diet, whether it be paleo or raw vegan. The answers I needed were often right in front of me and only required me to slow down the rational mind, but I consistently overlooked them, as I didn't know how to connect with my intuition or why I should in the first place.

I know I'm not the only one who has chosen thought over instinct in making choices in their life and with their food. Our experience today with food is drastically different than ever before in our evolutionary past, and I believe this is causing health problems. This concept goes far beyond the foods we're eating, once again; it has everything to do with the experience surrounding the food.

In our past, we embraced calories because starvation and survival were pressing concerns. Today, fewer people are concerned with starvation (but unfortunately many still are). If you're reading this, you likely have exponentially more freedom, choice, and opportunity than you had just 100 years ago, and surviving an attack from a predatory animal is the least of your concerns. You can get food delivered, order "superfoods," buy imported foods, as well as attempt to eat locally. In some ways though, we have fewer choices. It's not like I'm going hunting with a tribe to find some elk right now. That sucks, but that would also take all day, and I wouldn't be writing this right now.

The survival instinct is a central component to our experience with food. It is also a reason why we have increased rates of obesity today; weight gain can often be a protection from starvation. This survival mechanism explains why a history of dieting predisposes us to obesity; [32] our bodies want to protect us, and obesity is often a response to that. In addition, having evolved to survive better has protected us in many ways from weight loss, but not from weight gain. It's why anorexia nervosa is the most fatal psychiatric condition;[33] our bodies do not like to starve. Starvation is simply not compatible with health or reproduction, the latter of which is suppressed with any restrictive diet.

With this survival instinct in mind, we learned to recognize which foods were good for us. We're going to use the same instinct throughout this book to identify which foods are best for us at any given moment. Long term, using logic and intuition simultaneously will likely provide better results than just using intuition alone. And pre-modern humans did use logic as well to inform their decisions. They may have made careful observations and ran simple experiments to figure out what foods were best for their health.

But it wasn't the same type of logic people use today, where a diet is like a solved puzzle. I'm sure pre-modern humans may have constructed theories about what to eat. I have no evidence that they did not. But what I do know is that traditional cuisines from around the world reflect a different relationship with food than the one most health-conscious people have today.

Pre-modern humans didn't always get it right either, so I will stop placing them on a pedestal. For optimal health we must embrace all options that work instead of clinging to one ideology, even intuitive eating. That being said, my ramblings about the pitfalls of relying on nutrition science to construct a healthy diet and why we should embrace intuition for that purpose instead, is over. I hope that despite being a bit angry with me, you're now interested in trying something new and perhaps a bit crazy.

It is now time to begin activating your intuition. Take a break, look at the sky, and get ready for your second exercise. Being mentally and emotionally fresh is important for each of our exercises.

Intuition-Building Exercise #2: Time Travel

For this exercise, we will perform a visualization. Read the following description and travel back in time with me to a mythical place where humans were connected to their environment and ate intuitively.

Think of yourself now not just as a human but rather as a mammal. Identify with your mammalian mind. Imagine yourself living sustainably in nature, in the year 200,000 BC in a warm climate. You hunt your own food (if male), traveling long distances on foot (with very light footwear). You're vigilant of your surroundings, paying close attention to signs of prey. You're listening to every sound in the vast wilderness, looking for marks in the ground, and know what the signs are of fresh meat. If the hunt is successful, you come back home with the animal, storing it for future use for the tribe.

You sleep when it's dark, don't have Snapchat or Facebook, and breathe fresh air every day. You walk barefoot much of the time, physically connected to the healing energy of the earth, which has been shown to reduce pain and inflammation. You send smoke signals to contact neighbors and plan get-togethers.

If you're a woman, you spend time with your children every day. You don't have a 9-5 job. You weave baskets, tend to matters in the home, brew tea, and enjoy the varied tasks involved with nurturing and caring for your loved ones.

You're part of a tribe. You may still have plenty of stress from neighboring tribes and people, food shortages, and other factors. But you dance and sing around the fire and have a sense of community to alleviate your stresses. Your food culture is rich; you have help preparing delicious meals from elders and young ones. You are connected to your food, your environment, your people, and the earth.

Your food is fresh; you planted it or hunted it. You know exactly where it came from. You also didn't wash your hands with anti-bacterial soap as you prepared the meal; your microbiome is thus extremely diverse (for this and many other reasons). There are no antibiotic-resistant strains of bacteria around.

There is no refined sugar in your diet. You will have honey on occasion. You'll have the honeycomb too. It's raw—not heated to high temperatures. The boys got it from a tree nearby. Unrefined carbohydrates from starches and a variety of grains fuel you. When you eat meat, you don't just eat a New York strip steak. You eat organ meats, make broths, eat the tongue, brain, cheek, etc., making use of the whole animal.

Although this scenario does not perfectly mimic conditions in a hunter-gatherer society, it's somewhat similar. (I have based this scenario off the Hadza hunter-gatherers in Tanzania based on a research study I read about their diverse microbiome, relative to Westerners, and their diet).[34]

Now close your eyes and let this vision sink in. Modify it to your liking to mimic the conditions of humanity in a safe, sustainably living tribe eons ago. Let the feelings seep through you. Breathe the air, smell the smells, and taste the food. Smile with your tribal family members, and connect to the earth as simply as you once did.

Now contrast this above scenario to modern living. You are living in 2018 AD in a major metropolitan city. It's exciting to be in a big city sometimes, but the anti-anxiety effect of trees and nature certainly isn't benefiting your life right now. You work forty hours a week, indoors. You sit on a chair and certainly aren't moving about as you would if you were a hunter-gatherer 200,000 years ago.

You live in an apartment five stories above the ground with a roommate. No benefits of earthing for you, unless you make a trip to the beach or touch the ground barefoot on weekends. You like to drink and socialize in your spare time, especially on a Friday night. You're single, and like the thrill of meeting new people, especially for romantic encounters. Before bed, you check your phone, allowing blue-wavelength light waves to enter your eye and reduce growth hormone and melatonin secretion.

You don't sing and dance around a fire with your family members, but you are having fun with your friends on a regular basis. Your social health is great. But your diet could be better. You eat at food trucks once a day at least, and don't have much time to prepare delicious meals. Some fruit and oatmeal for breakfast might be all you get if you're lucky. You even think Chipotle tastes good.

For dinner you have a balanced meal with some carbohydrates, meats, healthy fats, and vegetables, all of which you purchased from a grocery store. You don't farm, so your microbiome isn't as diverse as that of the pre-modern man or woman. There's no time for that though, and that's why you rely on caffeine to get you through your day. It's not the calmest life, but it's what you must do to for now.

You friend tells you about the Whole30, so you pick up at the bookstore and start reading it every day. It gives you a list of several things to do. You love being organized, working hard, making plans, and so this diet plan fits you perfectly. You're now cooking more food at home, and following the script. But it feels like a chore. You wonder why you have to *do* so much to be healthy. Why can't it just be a state of *being*?

Close your eyes again and sit on this vision. How differently do you feel? Breathe the air again, smell the smells, hear the noises, and just think about how your intuition differs in each scenario. Think about how your all aspects of your health could possibly be different in 200,000 BCE compared to the present. Note, I said different, not worse.

Do not feel bad about anything. You are already starting to connect to your intuition just by reading and processing these two different scenarios.

Now, the difference between the pre-modern diet and the modern diet isn't just in the food. The food eaten is tied intimately to the experiences. But the same food, tied to different experiences, will have different effects on one's health. Understand that health includes emotional wellbeing as well as physical health, both of which are connected.

Eating socially, alone, walking, stressed, in a rush, in a loud environment, in nature, after you've cooked the food yourself, etc., are all examples of experiences surrounding the eating of food. How do you intuit and think this affects the health benefits of a food? Do you think that isolating the foods from a healthy culture that is connected to their food and environment, as described earlier, can produce the same health?

Intuition is a trait all of us possess. The pre-modern human was just more connected on average than we are, because there are multiple forces dampening our intuition. Both the pre-modern and modern human may fail to follow intuition with food. The pre-modern human may have a food shortage for example, and ignoring the intuitive cry for food may enhance survival. If that person was constantly thinking about food, he or she may be less successful in finding it. It is more adaptive therefore to suppress appetite and increase energy expenditure through the release of stress hormones. Fasting in the short term also has tremendous health benefits—thanks evolution!

And on the converse, the modern human may be very intuitive when it comes to food. This person may eat when he or she is hungry and stop eating when full. He or she knows how to eat things in moderation and avoid restrictive food rules. That person may not need this book, but will still benefit from learning to connect to food more deeply.

Fortunately, you don't have to drop everything and live in the jungle to follow your intuition, because it's a natural ability you already have. You just need to figure out how to use it. Start bringing awareness to your intuition right now as you keep reading and set the intention to awaken it, as in the next chapter, we will finally define it.

PART II

ENTER INTUITION

People mistakenly feel that the power to cure comes from outside themselves, administered by an alien intelligence.

—HARRIET BEINFIELD

3:
What Intuition Is and Is Not

A page from a journal of modern experimental physics will be as mysterious to the uninitiated as a Tibetan mandala. Both are records of enquires into the nature of the universe.

—FRITJOF CAPRA

THIS QUESTION CAN OPEN DOORS to a deeply philosophical debate. Not everyone agrees on what intuition is, but I have a very simple definition from my experience incorporating its advice over the past several years into my food, exercise, and lifestyle habits. **Intuition is a cognition-independent awareness of external (environment) and internal (body and mind) signals that relate to health, happiness, comfort, and/or survival.** By terming this 'cognition-independent' I'm implying that no thinking takes place. Intuitive awareness *comes* to us, consciously or unconsciously, allowing us to make an informed decision or take a guided action.

Intuition tells us what we want to eat, how we want to move and whatever else it is that we do. It will tell us if we can trust, date, befriend, or work with someone. Quite often, we may be unaware of the messages it is sending about the things occurring in our day-to-day lives. You can think of it as our inborn ability to "sniff" stuff out.

Intuition is often confused with educated guessing. Educated guessing involves relying on what one has already learned to make a prediction. Intuition on the other hand involves allowing information to come to us, rather than relying on what we have seen and heard before. Intuition does not involve thinking, planning, reasoning, or furrowing of the eyebrows (that's what I do when I think about a challenging problem or situation). In many ways, intuition is the complete opposite of thinking. Intuitive knowledge once again *comes* to us, as if flowing through us at whim; whereas, knowledge derived from thinking is *arrived* at, after careful methodical reasoning.

Consider the experience of medical intuitive Caroline Sutherland. Caroline worked in the field of environmental medicine for several years, and claims that one day, after arriving early to work, a bright light illuminated the back of the room. It got brighter and brighter until an angelic being of sorts came out of it and asked her if she will do "their" work. These types of mystical experiences are difficult to believe, but they are not uncommon.

Directly after this conversation, she began to see auras around all her patients and much more. She recounts the experience[35]:

> From then on, all I had to do was see a patient's name on a chart and I would immediately receive a flood of information about their treatment—which compounds to use, exactly where to start each treatment remedy, and anything else that was important to know…I would hear a distinct voice guiding me guiding me to items that didn't even appear on test forms…I could pick up a bottle of vitamins and *know* whether it would be effective for the patient, and what the dosage would be and how long the substance was required to be taken.

Caroline believes that she was contacted by a holy spirit. Although this experience sounds too mystical to be true, what catches my interest the most is the notion that she is able to intuit what therapies her patients needed. She is not alone in being a medical intuitive and being able to access vast amounts of information about a patient simply from reading their name or seeing their picture. Other examples of renown medical intuitives include Caroline Myss author of "Anatomy of a Spirit," and Anthony William of Medical Medium. If we were all able to do this, healthcare would be a lot different obviously. It may sound too good to be true, but I believe this is a rare ability that some people possess. The point is that intuition comes to us.

Another important difference between intuiting and thinking is speed of transmission. Thinking requires several parts of the brain working together simultaneously. Many neurons are involved; and although this process happens fairly quickly, intuition is faster. My theory as to why intuition is so much faster is based on the principle of nonlocality in quantum physics. Nonlocality implies that a particle exists everywhere at every time. It may show up at one identifiable location, but it exists far beyond just where it can be observed with the naked eye.

Assuming that consciousness carries matter, and that thoughts affect the universe physically, there is rationale to support the notion that with our intuition we can detect subtle changes in vibrations, consciousness, and matter. This conversation requires much more study, and is detailed further in "The Holographic Universe" by Michael Talbot. [36] Many of my experiences have been corroborated by the notions set forth in that book.

The principle of nonlocality may explain why when you think of someone close to you, what may actually be happening some of the time is that they thought of you first, and the thought was transmitted to your consciousness fairly immediately. This idea may explain how long-distance reiki, where the practitioner can send healing energy to a patient without requiring them to be physically present in the same room, works, if you buy that it does of course (I do). Although the experiments in quantum physics aren't conclusive enough to support that hypothesis, the work demonstrating nonlocality of quantum particles has inspired many people to jump on this bandwagon of thought, including myself.

Let me share with you a brief story. A close and very adventurous friend of mine decides to go hiking alone in the late fall. He takes a trail that is not on the map. It's colder than expected and parts of the trail are iced over. Navigating in the dark is quite difficult, so he decides to camp out for the night. My friend is a built man who enjoys braving the storms, but he is not prepared for the freezing temperatures. His body, tough as it is, complains about the cold, and he begins to shiver uncontrollably.

Eventually, he fears death—for the first time in his life—but remains calm. In the middle of the night now, his father, in another part of the country and not even aware that his son was in a life-threatening situation, wakes, bolting up in his bed, nervously thinking about his son's safety. He goes back to sleep, and later hears the story.

How is this possible? It's very tempting to see one possible solution and confirm it with our worldviews. I do not intend to convince you that my friend sent an energy signal to his father in the middle of the night due to quantum physics like Deepak Chopra would. However, I do believe it. How could my friend's father wake up nervously in the middle of the night as his son was near the brink of death by just coincidence? It makes more sense to me that we can transmit energies than the notion that these types of events are always due to random chance.

Perhaps you've had similar experiences. What I've observed is that when situations get dire, the chance of energetic communication taking place increases. Our intuitive ability is the metaphorical antenna that picks up this information. Our ability to understand that we are receiving messages with this antenna depends on our degree of mindfulness, awareness, and the amount of practice we've put into developing this innate ability.

As ridiculous as it may sound, perhaps there is more to the mind than the trillions of neurons hosted in our skulls. I gave this idea no merit when I first heard it until I began to experience intuition on a deeper level in my life, and came across more stories such as that of my friends.' Perhaps there are other parts of the brain that can explain the strange phenomenon intuitive understanding can give us (like thinking about someone right before they call you), but I have not come across any convincing explanations just yet.

The experiences reported by shamans and those who have ventured on a shamanic path of study also have a lot to say about intuition's role in understanding, well, life. South American shamans claim that by drinking a hallucinogenic brew known as ayahuasca, they are able to discern the medicinal properties of plants by communicating with them directly. I learned about this in Peru years ago, and my instructor on the trip told me that when she was under the influence of ayahuasca, one plant in particular called to her during the trip.

She ventured into the jungle to find it, and once she did, was surprised, as this plant wasn't known as a medicinal plant; it was just an ordinary plant that called to her for no apparent reason. It probably wanted attention as this study abroad trip was focused on learning about medicinal plants, and perhaps we've glorified medicinal plants because of single chemical constituents (active ingredients).

Beyond the seemingly ridiculous notion of plant-to-human communication, accounts from independent groups of shamans tell a consistent story about the origins of life, that if true, challenges academia's epistemic beliefs. Jeremy Narby suggests in his book "The Cosmic Serpent" that shamans may have known about DNA thousands of years before it was isolated in a laboratory by Watson and Crick.[37]

Narby discovered consistent patterns in the art work of South American shamans as well as that of Australian aborigines. In these drawings, he observed clear depictions of ladders, spiral staircases, double-helixes, serpents, and structures resembling chromosomes in various phases of the cell replication cycle. What seemed the most consistent were myths about the origins of life. In these myths, shamans describe serpents, often coiled around each other in a double helix, as the bearers of life.

One painter and ayahuascero (someone who performs ayahuasca rituals) who inspired Narby's work, Pablo Amaringo, possessed a photographic memory, which he used to recreate the visualizations he experienced on ayahuasca. In his drawings, Narby saw molecular biology: chromosomes in various stages of the cell replication cycle and double-helixes. In shock, Narby felt he had discovered something incredible.

Could ayahuasca have given shamans knowledge *directly*? I can't say for certain, but perhaps ayahuasca allows us to tap into knowledge that we normally cannot access. If that's truly possible, I have to seriously question why I ever opened a textbook to memorize material for an exam. Whatever the case, the point I'd like to illustrate is that knowledge need not be obtained just from scientific studies and logical thinking and reasoning abilities. There may be other mechanisms that are difficult for us to wrap our heads around that allow us to access factual information.

There are a variety of ways through which we receive intuitive insight. But what matters for our aim to eat intuitively is that intuitive insight comes directly to us, seemingly falling into our lap straight from the sky. Intuitive knowledge is just "there," waiting for our antennas to receive it. Once our antennas are working right, the intuitive insights flow into us, giving us the sense that we know something, without knowing the exact details just yet. Highly intuitive people act on this knowledge immediately, and may have more details to reveal than the untrained or less-intuitive. Those trained to think, like me, usually ignore this insight or take more time before acting on it. Once we learn to feel, we will be able to receive intuitive insight regularly.

The boldest claim I'll make about intuition, is that it's *always correct*. Intuitive insight may be incomplete, but it is correct, because it's based on real-world events and frequencies reaching us. It's an extreme statement, and from a scientific point of view, it's a fallacy to suggest something so boldly, but based on my experiences and research (which hasn't been a life-long investigation just yet), intuitive insights we get are more accurate than theories we come up with in our head from circular logic or faulty reasoning.

The difficult part in understanding this, again, has to do with how some might define intuition. Intuition has a very specific definition in my book. It can come in many forms, and it may have different mechanisms, but it is entirely different than thinking. Often, the mind may be silent when intuitive insight arises. At other times, it makes no difference. But it's something we are meant to know how to detect, and it is certainly one tool that can help us eat the way we're meant to again.

Sometimes, we may confuse intuition with thinking. We may think that our ex is trying to reach us for example because we are still attached to them. This is not intuition. I still am not a master yet in following my own intuition, so I still have moments where I confuse intuition with thought. But this is not unexpected, as the majority of my living experience was not conducive to training my intuition. But with time and practice, we get better at separating intuitive insights, which provide a glimpse of the truth, from our minds running on autopilot.

In contrast with intuition, thinking often follows a predictable path. We form associations between various ideas, sum up the evidence, and connect the dots together. This strategic method of reasoning is quite useful, but with food, unnecessary. Intuition is as predictable as nature is (unpredictably predictable). When something is out of balance, you can expect your intuition to tell you something. When things are in harmony, your intuition will tell you that everything is safe and sound.

The final difference between intuition and thinking for our purposes here, and one reason why it's easy to ignore intuition, is that it often operates in the background. We may not be clear on what intuition is always saying, because in the foreground, we pay attention to what we're doing in the present moment, or thinking about. One advantage however to this is that you don't actually have to pay attention to it.

It is just there, and when it signals, you will know—this takes practice to start seeing. Initially, you may have no idea where your intuition is! Thus, my goal for you with this guide is to give your intuition a microphone, elevating it from a tiny speck in the background, to having a place in the foreground, until it has a steady role in your life and you can consistently follow it when need be.

Applying Intuition to Eating

How can we apply this knowledge to how we eat? After all, there biological mechanisms that explain hunger, involving hormones such as neuropeptide Y, leptin, ghrelin, and signals from gut microbiota. But just like nutrition science, we don't really need to know this to understand how and when to eat. Thus, intuition with food may be explained by neurobiology, as well quantum physics.

We know when we're hungry. That's an example of intuitive insight, but we could argue that this hunger is mediated partly by hormones. However, what about different types of hunger? How can hormones explain specific types of hunger, like a craving for pickles, which I sometimes have? I don't know, yet, but I do believe that as you bring awareness to your body by implementing the *HYMTE* approach you will gain a better understanding of dealing with these specific types of cravings.

The difference between the biological basis for hunger and the intuitive cry for hunger has to do with wholeness vs. reductionism. In biology, we are required to reduce things to their parts to understand what causes what. To understand how ghrelin even works, we would have to understand its consequences when it's absent. The ensuing experimental model then uses mice, genetically engineered to lack this hormone.

After that, we may study humans with rare inherited disorders lacking this hormone. As explained previously, although these puzzle pieces may be valuable sources of knowledge, we can often screw up when we base our ideas on what to eat from different puzzle pieces. What typically happens when we apply reductionism to food is that something goes out of balance, there are side effects, and there are always new puzzle pieces we realize we forgot to put together. Intuition in contrast cannot be reduced to its parts. We can make sense of it, but it is one whole signal.

Thinking can and should certainly aid our intuition in constructing a healthy diet. If we lived before modern times, where water and seafood were not contaminated, and highly processed low-nutrient foods did not exist, then we could rely mostly on intuition to understand what to eat. But since this is not the case, exercising some rational judgment to the items on our plate can help us choose foods which serve us best, based on their chemical composition, growing conditions, pesticide applications, and other factors that influence our health.

However, our intuition should in theory always confirm our thinking. After formulating our hypotheses, our intuition can confirm whether or not they are true by telling us how we feel. I had a theory for instance that Nutella would improve my energy and metabolism. I ate a lot of it, and some of the symptoms I experience from stress seemed to decrease. But after a while, I started to feel inflamed. My throat felt uncomfortable, and my intuition told me to stop eating it. Two weeks went by, and I ate it again. The same thing happened. My body didn't like it.

But I persisted; I tried it again and I felt good again, until I didn't one last time. What I discovered about Nutella was that the high concentration of sugar does have a nice stress-alleviating benefit, but I do tend to feel inflamed. My joints even felt more stiff the days after Nutella, and since this affects my workouts, I threw out the tub, which had a lot of Nutella left. It took me a whole day to throw it out, I'll admit.

I honestly don't fully know what intuition is, or even when exactly it's working. But over the years, I've learned to apply intuition to my food choices, and it has improved my health. I've learned to apply it to my life, and it's resulted in better and quicker decisions. But I do have to be proactive about it because it's very easy for me to get lost in thought and ignore intuition.

I do believe that intuition can explain strange phenomenon, like when you start thinking of a friend seconds before they message you. We often label those experiences as coincidences, but what if our thoughts carry vibrations, and this can be communicated to someone else? In that case, it seems like less of a coincidence and more like a reality that our universe operates on. There's something about intuition that's a lot different than the way we're taught to think in school. Intuition is not part of course curricula, but it's part of our nature.

In sum intuition is the following:

- A cognition/thinking-independent awareness of external and internal signals that relate to health, happiness, comfort, and survival.

- A signal/message/insight that comes to us seemingly out of nowhere.

- Faster than thinking.

- Holistic: it cannot be reduced to its parts.

- Often operating in the background.

- Is always correct.

It's now time for our third intuition-building exercise.

Intuition-Building Exercise #3: Focused Meditation

Your third exercise involves a meditation, but not just any meditation. In general, meditation will enhance your intuition by reducing chatter and quieting the logical mind. This is highly recommended to do on a regular basis as you begin eating intuitively.

But the meditation exercise you're about to learn involves connecting deeper to intuitive insight about particular situations, people, and anything else that is relevant to your current life. Here is the procedure for this exercise:

1. Identify something important in your life right now. It could be your experience with a person, event, or even object. If you'd like, you can make it food-related too, but preferably not as we will practice more exercises specific to food later. What matters for this exercise is that it's something important or interesting in your life. Think drama, conflict, and emotionally charged-situations. If you experienced something recently that's on your mind concerning a person in particular, then choose that experience. If it's something food-related, choose that. It doesn't matter what it is.

2. Get into a meditation posture, with your legs crossed, in half-lotus, or full lotus. Sit on a meditation cushion if you have one, or on the *edge* of a seat with your feet on the ground, with no support for your back. Keep your back relaxed (no need to force it to be straight) and place your hands on your knees. Keep your eyes open for now until you read the rest of this procedure, but we will eventually close the eyes.

3. Take a few deep breaths to get centered and prepared for this exercise. Being emotionally prepared for what we do enhances productivity.

4. Now, bring up that person, event, situation, or thing that is on your mind.

5. As you visualize this situation, instead of *not* processing it at all, as is typical in meditation, we are going to go deeply into the experience with feeling. Observe any and all thoughts, sensations, judgments, and feelings that come up with regard to this situation. Make a mental list of what you're feeling and now pick one of them to explore deeply.

6. With this one feeling, sensation, judgment, or thought in mind, explore why it's there. By explore, I mean, visualize it. Feel that feeling. Think that thought, but don't get unfocused and wander. Stay on that particular train of thought and/or feeling. You may find that new insights to the situation arise. You'll hopefully start seeing it in a new way as you become aware of aspects of this situation that were not immediately noticeable before.

Don't worry if nothing comes up at first. Intuition takes some time to build. But once you get the hang of this meditation, you will likely be able to see things in new ways. The reason we're doing this exercise is because some of those feelings, sensations, and judgments are intuitive insights. Remember when we discussed how intuition *comes* to us? This type of meditation helps things come to you. And that's why it's not bad to be "judgmental" as some say. It's natural. When we learn to understand where that judgment is coming from we can learn a lot about the situation and even ourselves.

Feel free to jot down your thoughts, but it is not necessary. Once you experience the feeling, you will remember what to do about it. We may feel the compulsive need to write everything down lest we forget, but I think it is overvalued. Process the emotion inside your body. Once it sinks in, it's now with you and you have changed your frequency

4:
What My Cravings Taught Me about Deficiencies and What a Healthy Diet Truly Is

Perhaps we are so deeply habituated to believe that we can see only through our eyes that even in the physical we have shut ourselves off from the full range of our perceptual capabilities.
—MICHAEL TALBOT

I WANT TO SHARE SOME of the logical ways of dieting I subscribed to before eating intuitively. For many years, I applied logic to my food with intense devotion. Once I noticed that my health wasn't where it should be, I started to question my methods; I still questioned them logically however. It was only when unexplained phenomenon happened that involved intense feelings surrounding eating food did I begin to understand the role of intuition in helping me make food choices. I consequently also began to understand the role of intuition in making life choices more broadly.

I started my dietary journey with a low-fat diet to lose some weight to improve my performance on the high school track team. It made some sense. We have fat; so, if we eat less of it, somehow our own fat should disappear. While I ate my mini-wheats with skim milk for breakfast, I read the nutrition label on the cereal box. I was bored I guess.

After one-week of checking my abdomen and chest in the mirror multiple times daily, I ditched low-fat as I saw no results. I also didn't enjoy what I was eating. I liked fat and felt that the mini-wheats with skim milk was incomplete. I was now ready to embrace a new ideology to take me to my destination of the perfect body. I also quickly learned from my obsessive internet research that eating less fat wasn't a sound approach. In fact, our bodies turned carbohydrate into fat really, really well. Uh-oh. New rabbit hole discovered.

Before I go any further, I must share my motivation for going through these dietary trials. At the heart of many people's restrictive dieting habits is some burning desire to change something. If this desire for change comes from an unhealthy place, we may make decisions in haste. And the fragmented way we view nutrition is quite conducive to repeatedly making hasty decisions without ever seeing a bigger picture.

My story began at the age of 12 with the understanding that my body shape was abnormal. I have gynecomastia (gyno for short), a condition commonly known as man boobs. Man boobs however aren't always classifiable as gynecomastia. Sometimes they're just an overflow of adipose tissue on the chest that flap around as the person moves. In gynecomastia, man boobs are caused by a benign enlargement of glandular tissue,[38] due to an imbalance in the sex hormones.[39] This glandular tissue is much firmer than adipose tissue and doesn't flap around so much.

My pediatrician told me it usually goes away, and he was right. It's transient in most adolescents who develop it, lasting less than a year.[40] I prayed that that would be me, but it wasn't the case. The gyno persisted and I developed a fairly strong discomfort with my physique throughout my teens. I began to look forward to the cold Boston winters so that I could cover up the protruding pyramidal shape of my chest with some extra layers. But it always seemed to stand out when I scrutinized it.

The imbalance between testosterone and estrogen led to prominent roles of fat on my abdomen as well. I knew something wasn't right. This spawned my interest in being "healthy." I joined the track team in high school to lose those damn fat rolls. It worked, a little bit, but the gyno didn't change one iota. I palpated it every single day, and I felt absolutely no change despite seeing a visible reduction in abdominal fat. That's when it dawned on me to change my diet, and I began that brief trial with low-fat. But that didn't help either.

Shortly thereafter, I picked up a philosophy that has never left me. Natural. Organic. The way things are *meant* to be. But there really is no *meant*. Even the title of this book is deceiving. It just sounds good so I hope you'll forgive me. We *have* eaten a certain way for a long time, that is far different from the way we eat now, and it has many benefits. Less catchy than *meant*, I know.

The idea of being natural fascinates the perfectionist. I wanted my diet to be as perfectly natural as possible. Somehow, this led me to embark on a raw vegan diet. My goal was to get to 6% body fat. I thought that if my body fat was low enough, the gyno would change. I knew that the glandular tissue underneath my nipples was not adipose tissue and thus may not be modifiable through diet and exercise, but I stubbornly persisted.

On this diet I constructed an impressive series of logical arguments to support why it was healthy. Most people would likely agree that eating only fruits, vegetables, nuts and seeds is not healthy. But, my argument was that fruits contained as much protein as breast milk—about 5-6% by calories—and thus was sufficient for meeting my protein needs. I also believed that meat caused cancer and heart disease, constructing various arguments to support my beliefs. I quickly however found opposing points of view, which I acknowledged, open to the possibility I was wrong. Constructing a set of beliefs to support one's point of view isn't all that difficult I realized after several years, after doing it so fervently for a period of time.

I also read up on hormonal imbalances that could have caused my condition. Aromatase is an enzyme that converts testosterone to estradiol. Bodybuilders praised aromatase inhibiting substances for building muscle mass. Perhaps I needed to do the same. I wasn't willing to experiment with drugs, but I attempted to eat in a way that inhibited aromatase. I purchased various supplements that inhibited the enzyme, like chrysin, a compound found in honey. They didn't work, so I aimed to simply raise my testosterone levels naturally. Little did I realize that calorie restriction and overexercising increase cortisol levels, too much of which reduce testosterone.

Like any enzyme in the body, or any set of interactions between substances in the body, a delicate balance must be maintained. Men with aromatase deficiencies may have a low libido, low bone mass, and a range in testicular size from too small to too large.[41] Imbalance is a pain in the nuts apparently.

On the raw vegan diet, my body fat declined but my gynecomastia did not change at all. I was still palpating my glandular mass daily, until I heard that this could release prolactin. So I stopped, based on theories. I don't know why I was even afraid of prolactin as all hormones have complex roles in our bodies. I thought it was a feminine hormone (wrong). At least I *almost* had a ripped six-pack. There was still some abdominal fat that prevented my abs from being picture-worthy, in my troubled mind.

After the raw vegan diet, which I committed to for thirteen months, I became fascinated with carbohydrate restriction. I also developed an intense craving for cheese, the strongest food craving I have ever experienced in my life. This craving occurred a few months after ending the diet. Sometimes our intuition gets so blocked from the humdrum of our lives that we don't realize what we really need.

I wasn't vegan anymore, but I was still somewhat attached to the habits that I created on the raw vegan diet. Every day for thirteen months I ate massive amounts of fruits and vegetables—it became a habit. Many of my meals were still raw vegan meals, which had me chewing and chewing away, for way too long. But I had to investigate this craving. I went to an organic market in the college town I lived in and purchased two solid chunks of cheese, both square-shaped. One was off-white in color and the other was a very light shade of yellow.

The following account may sound unbelievable, but I assure you it's 100% true. I took one bite, just one bite of the cheese, without any condiments whatsoever. I was waiting for the bus and eating this cheese while standing. I don't recall exactly how long it took for the cheese to hit my brain, but it was a matter of minutes. I became intensely euphoric. My mood shifted from where I was normally at, just an unremarkable average mood, to a state of limitless possibility. I felt more energy in my muscles as well and thought about sprinting as far as I could without stopping.

In the moment, I started laughing, thinking about how amazing life is. I wanted to high-five everyone I saw, but there was no one around at this bus stop. The best part was, I ate the entire block of cheese and an additional few bites from the next block. I inhaled roughly one-thousand calories in ten to fifteen minutes. The euphoric effects plateaued early on however, roughly at around a few ounces of cheese, but my appetite craved roughly ten ounces. I was high as shit.

I wondered what it could have been in the cheese that boosted my mood and energy so much. Was it saturated fat, calcium, the small amounts of omega-3s, or something else? It was most likely all of those things, and especially the large dose of saturated fat. From a physiological perspective, it's hard to imagine that the cellular processes that got upregulated after I ate all that cheese could have done so in just minutes. There is most likely a scientific explanation that I'm not exactly sure of even to this day. However, I have a "big picture" theory that attempts to explain not just this phenomenon, but a lot of problems people encounter with dieting.

It's incredibly simple. Restriction of any kind takes away life, and abundance gives life. Restriction seems like a sensible approach to limit something very good: something that could easily become too much of a good thing. Sex, sugar, fat, and alcohol are examples. Let's focus on sugar. An abundant quantity of refined sugar you may argue is not giving us more life; it's doing the opposite, and thus contradicts my theory.

But an abundance of refined sugar in the diet involves restriction in other ways. Cane sugar for instance still has antioxidants, whereas refined sugar has little to none. Fruits have sugar as well as minerals, vitamins, fiber, and phytonutrients, and is in a sense far more 'abundant' than high quantities of refined sugar. As is often the case, an abundance of refined sugar in the diet usually means that there is some imbalance. Someone consuming 25% of their caloric intake from refined sugar for example may not be getting enough protein and nutrient-dense foods. But on the converse, eating *only* foods that are "abundant" sources of sugar like fruit may be restrictive too, especially for an athlete with a high workload.

In this sense, even the standard American diet could be a restrictive diet, or at least have parallels to it, for being an abundant source of sweet, salty, and fatty foods. Since this "restriction" happens inadvertently and from the overconsumption of nutrient-deficient foods, deficiency is a more accurate term. Restriction is usually a deliberate action. The SAD is *deficient* in bitter, pungent, astringent, and sour tastes, among many other things.

Whether this deficiency happens deliberately from restriction or by consequence of overconsumption of highly palatable and addicting foods, it results in us feeling less *alive*. When you imagine feeling alive, what do you see? I see smiles, sunlight, low stress, and freedom. That's what I experienced from eating cheese after a long period of restriction. And I never craved cheese like that again, or experienced such intense euphoria from eating something.

Sugar Saves Lives

For about three to four years I abstained from sugar, excluding naturally occurring sugars in fruit. When I was raw vegan I ate massive amounts of fructose, but I boycotted fruit juices, thinking I was more natural in some sense. The first sugars I began adding in my diet a couple years after that experiment included honey and sugars from milk (lactose). But it was not until four years after I began my experiment with raw veganism when I finally let go of my fear of gaining fat and embraced added sugars from *drinks*.

At this point, I had been training like a maniac in the gym for five years or so, in the attempt to increase my vertical jump to 42 inches, so that I could dunk a basketball. My training and my diet consumed me. If I ate normally I probably would have gained strength more quickly, but my perfectionist attitude caused me to eat restrictively. Eventually fatigue set in my body on a daily basis. My eyes felt tired, like they wanted to close. During the day, I meditated a lot, just to close my eyes. In classes I fell asleep early on in lecture. My attention was not as intense and didn't last as long. These problems began on the raw vegan diet, but my training in combination with undereating most likely exacerbated the problem.

I learned about a blog called 180degreehealth,[42] run by a man who had also been through similar dietary experiments. He hiked through mountains and dieted extremely only to find that his metabolism started to slow. The addition of processed junk foods to his diet reversed all those abnormalities and restored him to health. He thus advised the restrictive eater to eat more junk food, not only to raise metabolism, but to combat disordered eating habits that get ingrained deep in our psyches. His advice certainly was controversial.

I learned that I had many of the symptoms of a low metabolism that Matt described. I was getting cold more often, was fatigued, and my body temperature was in the 97's, which was too low. The outer third of my eyebrows were sparse, which is a symptom of hypothyroidism. The most concerning symptom were the gray hairs I developed around the side of my scalp. Being in my early twenties, I knew there was a problem. So after reading his blog for a while I decided to eat sugar. Evil, evil sugar. Having gray hairs and mild chronic fatigue was far worse than eating some sugar at this point.

It was surprising to me that avoiding added sugar, salt, and processed foods could be unhealthy. But it was time to change my opinions because I had accepted finally that I was missing something really important.

I found an "organic" soda made with evaporated cane sugar, sat down at the café I regularly went to and took a sip. Have you ever been stupid enough to walk 30 miles across a desert without drinking any water? Didn't think so. I haven't either, but just imagine what tasting water would feel like after walking for eight hours in the heat with just your camel but no water. It would taste amazing. You wouldn't even care if it was tap water contaminated with xenoestrogens. You'd just care that it hydrated your cells.

As if I was parched for several years, this sugary drink tasted like heaven. From the first sip, I felt my brain light up. The pleasure and reward centers of my brain celebrated. I went on to drink three of them a day for one week, then slowed down to about one a day for perhaps a month. Eventually my cravings for this soda vanished, and my energy improved. My eyebrows looked fuller and I felt better overall.

My intuition didn't know it craved soda. I had to read about how it could possibly help me, try it out myself, and observe the results. The reason why this sugar craving didn't magically come to me like the cheese craving did is because intuition can get suppressed. Activating it and learning how to use it will be described in the following chapters.

Learning that sugar improved my health and made me feel less stressed and more energized taught me to start following my gut rather than the theories I read about in the scientific literature and from low-carb gurus.

What Cheese and Sugar Ultimately Taught Me

The cheese I ate increased my body's perception of energy availability and abundance. The metabolic processes in my body that were stagnant got turned on. If I had an abundance of mood and metabolism-boosting neurotransmitters in my brain already, eating all that cheese wouldn't have taken me to supraphysiologic levels, as our bodies try to keep things in balance. The feeling eating that cheese gave me was all the evidence I needed to conclude that whatever diet I was previously on was not life-giving, but highly restrictive. This may seem obvious to some of you, but I was convinced that my raw vegan diet supplied everything I needed for optimal health.

These examples of cheese and sugar elevating my metabolism involve some complicated physiology. Let's simplify it and look an extreme example. We can all agree that starvation is not good for us. Deliberate attempts at eating less food despite the body's objections leads to lower levels of sex hormones, increased food cravings to the point of obsessive thoughts about food, and a decreased metabolic rate.

These effects are not life-giving, in that they put a halt to energetically expensive processes like reproduction. Someone affected by starvation clearly looks unhealthy and weak. The solution here is to provide adequate calories, from any source. The longer the restrictive dieter waits to take in extra calories, the longer it may take to fully recover.

Once I "gave in" to foods that I had once restricted, my health returned to close-to-normal. What do I need to do to get back to a stellar state of high metabolic energy on most days? Manage my stress, by eating regularly, exercising only when I feel energized enough, put extra effort in my recovery, deep breathing and gentle yoga, and proper sleep.

School affected several of these variables, but since that episode is now over, I can take on recovery full-throttle again. Compared to the days where logical ideas of what to eat dominated my choices, my energy, metabolism, and mood is far better now. I've now learned to eat when I feel like I need to, for my overall health, versus eating from a set of rules.

Rules

Dietary rules are one hallmark of the logical eater that we must address before learning about how we're meant to eat. These rules ultimately exist to back up a philosophy. When I was raw vegan, I believed that fruit contained as much protein as breast milk and therefore was actually an adequate source of protein as long as I met my minimum caloric requirements. I thus ate massive amounts of fruit but never got the same *satisfaction* I got from meat once I started eating it again. I learned that this belief didn't lead me to feeling as great as actually eating highly absorbable sources of protein like animal foods, and slowly learned to ditch it. This happened though trial and error, rather than by finding a new logical food rules to replace the old ones.

As a reminder, intuitive eating has a zero-tolerance policy for your beliefs about what is healthy and what isn't healthy. Most people will thus find it extremely challenging. Believing in an ideology is paramount to the success of a diet. All diets are based on belief systems that are supported with skewed logic. A diet must have clueless fans who are willing to vouch for its efficacy. I used to be one, and maybe you are too, but not anymore after this chapter. You are now belief-less, and open to new possibilities. You are ready to acknowledge that your body may have an interest in a food item that you thought was unhealthy, but is not anymore, because your body needs it. You are ready to move on from beliefs and begin to accept the truths your intuition is informing you about.

In the next chapter we will discuss how beliefs and other factors may be blocking your intuition and perform an exercise to understand our beliefs. Your requirement for this exercise is to be honest with yourself. Take a breath, go outside, and start increasing your self-awareness. It's going to be fun, once you learn to flow.

5:
Common Factors Blocking Intuition

...gazing out the train window at a random sample of the Western world, I could not avoid noticing a kind of separation between human beings and all other species. We cut ourselves off by living in cement blocks, moving around in glass-and-metal bubbles, and spending a good part of our time watching other human beings on television.

—JEREMY NARBY

IMAGINE THIS COMMON SCENARIO. Melanie arrives at the CrossFit gym at 5:30 AM, despite being tired, because she's trying to lose weight, and well, because there's a workout every day (it's called the workout of the day, or WOD). She is an extremely motivated person, so it frustrates her that she's experiencing fatigue; she's fighting her body to get to the gym. As usual, she consumes a caffeinated pre-workout supplement before heading there. It doesn't work as well as usual, but nevertheless, she's focused on how her efforts will pay off later. Manifestation, right?

She's also craving carbohydrates, but since she's on the Paleo diet, she limits her intake quite a bit. By blatantly ignoring her intuition she is on her way to experiencing the ill effects of chronic stress. Say hello to accelerated aging and cellular damage. Her hair may begin falling out, her body temperature may drop a point, and her metabolism will become increasingly sluggish. Her intuition is constantly telling her to take rest and eat pancakes and maple syrup instead of bacon and eggs like she usually does, but she's not mentally ready to let go of her low-carb-paleo ideology yet.

Months go by, and now she is truly suffering. She is finally open to the idea that her regimen may be imbalanced to say the least. Her physical strength and endurance is decreasing. She feels stressed and knows that this can cause inflammation. She also knows that she's craving sugar, but suppresses those instincts. From my Instagram, she reads a post captioned "Anorexia nervosa is the most fatal psychiatric condition": starvation is not compatible with life. Below the post I discuss that this condition involves low bone density, decreased strength, and increased inflammation. She wonders for the first time now if her workouts, in addition to her low-carbohydrate diet, could be causing her symptoms. For the first time she asks herself: "am I exercising too much?" DING! She's now onto something.

Melanie is not alone. Each day, millions of people participate in some health activity because they read about it online or hear about it from their doctor even. Some people stick to these ideas for a long period of time, and others give up after a short period of time. Those that give up follow their instincts. Those that don't, follow their logical minds, unless it really makes them feel better.

Those who stick to the plan may see better health temporarily, but after a period of time, experience imbalances. It's human nature to not want to give up, which can worsen the imbalance. But it's not giving up here, it's about listening to your body.

There are a variety of factors that predispose people to not listen to their bodies. But before we talk about the intuition blocking factors, let's briefly define health, since that's our goal. My favorite definition of health comes from the homeopath George Vithoulkas.[43] He states:

> Health is freedom from pain in the physical body, a state of well-being; freedom from passion on the emotional plane, resulting in a dynamic state of serenity and calm; and freedom from selfishness in the mental sphere, having as a result total unification with truth.

I love this definition because it's qualitative, abstract, and makes sense to me with a variety of situations. For example, when you are pain-free, you are free to do things physically without pain. When your mind is healthy you have more freedom to interact with others, work, play, etc. When you have no injuries you are free. When you don't have any eating limitations you are free from tormenting thoughts on what to eat. In contrast, Melanie in our example was not free; she was restricted by the chains of a toxic belief system. The freedom in the mental plane will influence the physical plane, as health of the mind is connected to health of the body.

Once you learn to *identify* the intuition blocking factors in your life and then *remove* them, you will become freer, which will allow you to be more present with yourself, put yourself and your needs first, and embrace a new type of health.

I want you to first determine what the uniquely qualitative elements of health are for *you*. Hint: emotions play a role. Your enjoyment of life plays a role. And diet, movement, sunlight, grounding, fresh air, sexuality, and quality sleep plays a role in all of this. It's all connected. Take a few moments to write them down.

Now let me share mine. For me health is freedom but also a subjective experience. Having mental clarity, physical energy, flexibility, good joint lubrication (not feeling as stiff during yoga), being motivated, and being alert throughout the day are some aspects of health that I've learned to correlate with various lifestyle modifications. But even more qualitatively, and on a deeper level, when I'm at my healthiest, I have more ideas flowing in my mind. I feel more tolerant towards things that test my patience. I feel more at ease with everything. I'm also more energized and conversational with others. My empathy improves.

As you start to eat intuitively, I suggest writing down those subjective and qualitative health experiences that you feel are influenced by the foods you eat. After that, developing the habits to continue doing what's working and modify accordingly can keep you healthy in the way you have defined for yourself.

I believe that in a truly healthy state, one must be strongly in touch with their intuition. And when one is strongly in touch with their intuition, they have the power to achieve greater health, by understanding what's working and what isn't. It's a beautiful cycle.

Now, for a variety of reasons, many people aren't listening to their intuition at all. As you go through the list below, take a moment to pause after each listed factor and decide if this is relevant to your life. Reading isn't just about going through the words with your eyes. Comprehension, perception, understanding, confusion, then application are important elements of reading that help you understand the content. This requires more investment, energy, and time. You can use your own intuition to decide if that extra investment is worth it for you, based on how well this resonates. But I would suggest sitting on each intuition-blocking factor listed below to discern whether or not it's affecting your life. Are you ready to investigate the role of intuition-blocking factors in your health?

The Logical Mind

Goals. Achievements. Work. Tasks. Job. Completion. Failure. Success. All these words here cover one important reason why intuition goes unheard: the intellectual and logical mind. This pathway may become activated when we have tasks to complete, or, as in the example of the morning exerciser, goals to achieve. Maybe those goals stem from a belief system, like the inner voice telling the CrossFitter that carbohydrates are inherently fattening. When these thoughts penetrate our minds, intuition takes a time out.

The logical mind was the main reason why my intuition used to be suppressed.

Beliefs

When you have faith in an idea, true or not, we may call it a belief. I have a belief that intuition has changed the way I view the world over the past several years. I believe that many people completely ignore their intuition. I believe that intuition is absent from conventional healthcare. And I also believe that strong beliefs about diet and exercise are analogous to religion. Religions like Christianity, Islam, Hinduism, Judaism, and Buddhism involve *faith*. Having strong faith is seen as a good thing. In Hinduism, disciples are called devotees.

When I was on the raw food diet, I was essentially a devotee on some strange but hopefully fruitful path with other devotees. Our belief system was integral to our emotional and spiritual wellbeing. There was no room for contrary beliefs to enter our headspace. This is exactly how many devoutly religious individuals think. Devout vegans therefore seem to be practicing an organized religion.

Having strong beliefs doesn't have to be a bad thing. It's really the rigidity of those beliefs that can get us into trouble. I strongly believe that good food and natural medicines can treat most illnesses. But if I develop a life-threatening infection in the jungle that does not improve with natural means, I will opt for an antibiotic (last resort). There's a chance that I would be stubborn however and just die, but I if I'm in the jungle in the future I'll come prepared with immunity-boosting and antimicrobial herbs and obviously make sure to research what conditions I could be afflicted by.

When it comes to beliefs, it is best to be fluid, not rigid. This allows us to accept vital intuitive insights that can improve our lives.

Intuition-Building Exercise #4: Identify Your Food Beliefs

There are several other intuition-blocking factors left to discuss, but it's time for another exercise. Take a deep breath. Get up, stretch it out, and get some water. This exercise is **crucial** in your intuitive eating journey. *Beliefs* are one of the most significant intuition-blockers, and we can inherit them easily. The more impressionable you are, the more easily your diet will be influenced by a belief that is not your own. Imagine that! Beliefs are often implanted in our heads by alien life forms.

You may watch a TED talk for example and start to form a belief. Perhaps you've been following the advice of your favorite blog and this has impacted your beliefs. Or maybe you were scrolling through your phone at night without night mode switched on (how foolish of you!) and saw some post about "fit girls" and decided to eat an açai bowl the next morning to achieve a thigh gap. Or maybe you thought you need to cover all your electronic devices with blue-wavelength-light-blocking screen covers, and your health did not improve whatsoever. These are all beliefs that may or may not improve your health and the best way to find out is to experiment and be detached from them so you can let them go when the experiment fails.

Whatever the case, if your food beliefs come from anything other than your own personal experience with food, they must be destroyed for this exercise. You will now construct beliefs from scratch by following your own body and NOT the advice of anyone else based on logical theories.

Get out a sheet of paper or an electronic device that you can write on, and identify as many of your food beliefs as possible. Make a list or draw a mind map of sorts. I would recommend starting with a list to keep things simple, but try something that works for you. I'm a list guy, but occasionally I like making mind maps where I write down several ideas on different parts of the same page (on non-lined paper), and scribble freely in between, draw lines, and get more creative. Decide on your method of choice here, and spend at least 10 minutes on it.

This exercise shouldn't be completed in one sitting. You may have beliefs buried far back in your mind that you will only realize when you examine the way you add milk to your coffee (*ahem—I'm describing myself here. I realized I didn't add enough milk to my coffee to give it that creamy taste because I was afraid of adding too many calories to it. Once I made that realization, I said "fuck it" and added as much milk as I really wanted).

Identify at least **five** beliefs that play a role in determining what foods you eat on a daily basis. Then, as other beliefs pop into your head, add them to this list. The purpose of this exercise is just to *identify* those beliefs; it is not to deconstruct them—that will happen later. By writing them down, you will begin the process of deconstructing them anyway

Stress

Burden. Trapped. Constricted. Fight. Escape. Hate. Exhausted. There are many ways people describe being stressed. Exercise is even a form of stress. There are good stresses and bad stresses. Good stresses help you grow. Bad stresses bring you down. Accelerated aging and cellular damage result. Whatever type of stress it is, it will impede intuitive processes, through various mechanisms. One simple way it could do this is by preoccupying us, preventing us from being aware of what we need.

But stress can also awaken intuition. Determine now what kinds of stresses you are experiencing. There may be some good ones, and some not so good ones. Determine next if these stresses are affecting your relationship with food. Do this mentally, or write it down on that sheet of paper, or document it electronically. By the end of this book, you should have a nice document with several observations and intuitive insights you can learn from for a while.

Find gratefulness, love, acceptance, and forgiveness. Let go. Sit up straight and close your eyes. Notice your breathing become freer—not stifled and constricted. Practice some asanas (yoga poses) in the morning. Take a cold shower. Your mental state can change from developing a healthy relationship with a stress that maybe you've dealt with for a while. Perhaps you can walk away, in which case, you may experience more short-term stress before seeing a long-term benefit.

Whatever the case, for the purpose of awakening your intuition, practice bringing awareness to your stresses first. This includes how those stresses affect you. Feel it. Then figure out how to deal with them. It may sound obvious, but I think sometimes reading the obvious can really help.

Distractions

Snapchat. Netflix. News. Notifications. Messenger. Twitter. Neighbors. Family. Friends. There are a variety of distractions that can have us completely ignore our intuition. Perhaps you eat every single meal while streaming Netflix. How do you think this is affecting your intuition while you eat? Maybe you're eating past the point of being full. Maybe you're not even eating because you're hungry.

Identify, and then slowly remove the distractions. Establish healthy boundaries while being aware of what you need. You may not have to completely say no; you just have to adjust after becoming aware. Make a mental note or write down which distractions prevent you from connecting to your food and accessing your intuition.

Addiction

Alcohol. Sex. Drugs. Rock'n Roll. iPhone. Facebook. Android. Ipad. I once attended a family dinner where a young boy of three or four years old was so consumed by a game on the iPad he was unable to eat. His mother tried to feed him some rice and lentils, but struggled as he attempted to evade her, eyes glued to the device. Eventually, he played it smart and tried to create the semblance that he was complying, by messily stuffing some rice in his mouth, causing grains of rice to spill on his shirt, chair, and floor. The iPad had much greater control over him than his parents did.

This remarkable sight made me wonder. Would this boy's appetite be any different if he wasn't so consumed by the attention-sucking game on the device?

Most likely, yes. You see, there is a pathway in the brain that lights up when we do something we fancy. Drugs are a great example. They make people feel good, and this stimulates the reward pathway in the brain, which involves dopamine producing neurons in the nucleus accumbens and ventral tegmental area. When these neurons are stimulated, we will want to perform that activity again, even if it stops feeling as good after a while. This area can be electrically stimulated in rats to produce dopamine directly, by hooking up their dopamine-producing neurons to a lever.

In the 1950s, psychologists James Olds and Peter Milder found that rats would press this lever upwards of 1,000 times in an hour. If left to it, some would die of starvation. The four-year-old child I mentioned was having the same experience. The game was simply more exciting than food.

Many things may be more exciting than eating food, but to connect to your intuition, slowly remove them when you eat. Try eating one meal a day without any distractions. For the meals where you Netflix, read, check your phone, or add another rewarding activity to your meal, bring attention and mindfulness to your appetite.

Addictions and distractions can often overlap. You may experience them both in a single meal, causing your intuition's voice to drown in the gripping, controlling, desperate cries from the reward center. "Please me!" it will say. The abundance of dopamine-releasing and potentially soul-sucking activities at our fingertips makes it quite easy to please the reward center.[44]

Environmental Contaminants and Toxins

Bisphenol-A. Polychlorinated biphenyls. Organochlorane pesticides. Sodium lauryl sulfate. Triclosan. Aluminum sulfate. *Chemicals are everywhere*. They are inside of us, catalyzing important cellular processes, but also toxifying the oceans. Chemicals aren't all bad. In fact, glucose is a chemical. Chemistry is happening in your body right now because of the glucose in it.

Bisphenol-A is also a chemical. It's a bad one however, that is associated with increased diabetes risk[45] and many other conditions. The science isn't entirely clear, but in general, toxins can affect how our bodies perceive food. Exactly how, I don't know, and I don't really want to honestly. I've never been a huge fan of horror movies.

Intuition may not be able to detect what toxins are in your body. However, you can use intuition by attempting to cleanse for a period of time, fasting, and noting how you feel.

Toxins are best dealt with by thinking rather than intuiting. This book is not about how to detox, but chances are that you have various industry byproducts present in your adipose tissue,[46] bloodstream, breast milk,[47] and excrements. If you've been eating unmindfully for a period of time, preparing foods at home using organic and non-GMO ingredients may help facilitate detoxification, which may in turn improve intuition. Adding spices, hot yoga, sauna therapy, and detoxifying baths may also help in this regard.[48] However there is little research supporting the use of these protocols to detoxify environmental contaminants.

Altered Gut Microbiota

Clear patterns illustrate the difference in the gut between obese and inflamed individuals and lean and healthy individuals. We have over 400 species of bacteria in our gut, falling into five main families. Of those, two are the most predominant: *Bacteroides* and *Firmicutes*. Obese people see an increase in the ratio of *Bacteriodes* to *Firmicutes* relative to lean people.[49] These gut flora can increase inflammation, and make us crave weight-gain-promoting foods.[50]

Exactly how the obese develop this balance of microbiota is unclear, but it seems that the imbalance creates further imbalance. You'd think that you'd be able to tell when you're starting to fall out of balance, but it seems that it's not as simple as falling off a teeter-totter. Just like an alcoholic, the alcoholic craves alcohol when he doesn't need it. How do we shift the balance back?

The body must receive information to shift back to a healthy and normal state, with new input (change in diet). Rebalancing the gut microbiome is a subject that is beyond the scope of this book, but the point is that intuition can become confused from signals being sent from the gut bacteria. This may lead to eating behavior that is not necessarily what your body really wants, but what these invaders want. It's a fascinating subject and a relatively new area in the field of obesity and chronic disease and is just presented as food for thought here, no pun intended.

Regardless, the methods of intuitive eating that will be outlined shortly can work for those with an imbalanced gut microbiome. Once you try new foods and see how you feel, you can calibrate and adjust to achieve optimal energy, health, and subjective well-being.

Chronic Diseases

Many conditions fall into the category of chronic disease. Examples include diabetes, cardiovascular disease, multiple sclerosis, inflammatory bowel disease, rheumatoid arthritis, and many more. These pathologies can occur in those with inherited predispositions, but they are mostly cause by lifestyle, and unfortunately they affect people for years, if not decades. Whatever the case, there are a variety of them and they may influence your intuitive abilities. Whatever the case, intuition is always with you. If suppressed because of a disease, bring awareness to it to begin waking it up.

Poor Diet

Canola oil. GMOs. Refined sugar. Enriched wheat flour. Cereals. Soda. Fast-food. Yes, your diet is implicated in the above three intuition-hindering factors (environmental toxins, altered gut microbiome, and chronic disease). We eat daily, and the food we eat carries with it information that your entire body *remembers* afterwards. As the next chapter will explain, with a limited diet, you have limited information, and your intuition has less to choose from.

Someone who grew up on fast food in the deep South (Alabama, Georgia, Louisiana, Kentucky, Texas, Florida...the most obese states in America essentially) may not know what their bodies need to eat. They only know what they have been exposed to. Based on this assumption, a diet that lacks diversity makes it harder for your intuition to understand what it needs.

Just imagine being on a chronic high-sugar, high-fat, low-bitter (the taste) and low-fiber diet for twenty years. You go to the popular fast-food chains. You drink low-quality coffee. Perhaps you smoke cigarettes. If you do cook food, your vegetables aren't very fresh. Yes, it may sound frightening, or maybe it describes your own life or the life of someone you know. There is no diet cure for those who simply don't have the option to eat nutrient-dense food (even though we all should have that option, and it doesn't need to be expensive). Someone on this diet likely won't be craving turmeric. They are used to eating low-nutrient, high-calorie foods, without many antioxidants or disease-fighting properties.

To find balance, these people must add different foods to their diet. If all you know is fried chicken, French fries, fried Kool-Aid, and barbeque, your choices are limited by your memory. Heard of "acquired" tastes? Well you may need to acquire *new* tastes and connect with them to allow your intuition to tell you what it wants, especially if your diet has not been varied in the past.

Severing the Attachments

Between us and our connection to intuition lie any number of the above listed factors, and many other factors I did not include. They all prevent us from receiving intuitive insight. And most importantly, they're all reversible.

What we're going to do together is start noticing when intuition is being blocked—when eating, when working, when walking, or doing anything we normally do. We'll also tune into what is blocking it, how it's being blocked, and why it's being blocked. Once you start to see the why, when, where, and how, you can begin removing the obstacles in the way.

Now when it comes to intuitive *eating*, realize that there will be some uncertainty jumping into it. Intuitive knowledge doesn't seem certain to everyone, especially those trained to think about all their problems. If you've trained yourself to approach healthy eating from a logical basis, you may feel uncomfortable with not knowing exactly how many calories or carbohydrates you are consuming.

If you've ever subscribed to a certain dietary philosophy, such as the Paleo diet, the Whole30, or even my favorite, Weston A. Price (WAPF, or Weston A. Price Foundation, recommends consuming bone broths, raw and fermented dairy, cod liver oil, and organ meats, foods which seem to be consumed around the world by various traditional peoples and societies), you may feel conflicted with a belief you once had and your intuition's calling. I experienced this regularly when transitioning from a vegan diet to a low-carbohydrate Paleo diet, to a Weston A. Price diet, and to a more balanced diet.

For example, when I was on a Weston A. Price diet, I consumed a lot of raw milk. I thought it was an excellent food for health. I learned about the differences between pasteurized and raw milk. I lobbied for the legalization of cow shares in the capitol of Maryland, Annapolis (this would allow people to legally own a part of a cow, which was one way to obtain raw milk). I made smoothies out of it. I fed raw milk ice cream to my girlfriend at the time (whose intuition said it was just "okay," whereas my logical brain said it was awesome even though I knew that she was right). Raw milk became part of my life. It was attached to it.

I couldn't ignore however the observation that when I drank less milk, my throat was more clear. When I drank milk, I would have to clear my throat more. AHEM—ah—hum—gah. Furthermore, my voice simply wasn't as resonant and clear. When abstaining from milk, my voice was so clear I felt as if I could become a singer, so I became one and traveled to another universe but came back to write this.

Choosing between having uncongested vocal cords and drinking milk was not easy, but ultimately, I made the decision to cut milk from my diet for the rest of my life except in minimal quantities. I used almond milk in my coffee and tea for a period of time for instance, and enjoyed my beautiful voice when I spoke to myself in my studio apartment. But then, one day, I wanted milk again. So I drank it, and my vocal cords didn't get as clogged! I don't know what happened, but perhaps there was an *interaction* between milk and other factors in my diet (stress?) that caused me to have to clear my throat a lot. I now go through phases where I will drink cow's milk and others where I'll abstain from it.

Intuition-Building Exercise #5: Identify the Intuition-Blockers in Your Life

It's time to make a complete list of the factors that are blocking your intuition. Using the same sheet of paper you used for exercise #4 ("Identifying Your Food Beliefs"), create a 2x2 table. Title the left column "Intuition-Blocking Factors" and the right column: "How I Plan to Diminish Their Impact."

In the left column, list which factors mentioned in this chapter you feel are currently blocking your intuition. On the right side, jot down a phrase, a few words, or even a complete sentence or two to set the intention regarding how you plan to reduce the impact of this intuition-blocking factor with your eating habits.

Don't think too hard about this. Remember, intuition is a lightning-quick insight you get about something. It's the first thing that comes to you. You may be tempted to ignore it too. I still deal with this regularly, but have learned to acknowledge its existence in almost every instance.

PART III

METHODS OF *HYMTE*—STEPS TO EATING INTUITIVELY

Though this be madness, yet there is method in't.
—WILLIAM SHAKESPEARE

6:
Understanding How, Why, and When You Eat

WE ALL HAVE A FOOD STORY. We've developed relationships with food through our cultural backgrounds, upbringing, lifestyle, and other life experiences. These need to be sorted out through mindfulness, as our stories may dampen our intuition.

Consider for example Tony. He has trouble walking because of diabetes. Even reaching a standing position from the couch in his modest studio close to the beach is difficult. His condition is severe. In fact, his toes self-amputated due to a loss of blood flow. This degree of diabetes is truly life-threatening. One day, as I couchsurfed at his abode in southern California, he recounted his food story.

It involved his mother nagging him to finish eating dessert. He was already full, but acquiesced, just to please her—he couldn't say no to his mother. He grew up on fried food, fast food, sweets, and the exact type of diet that is implicated in the diabesity epidemic, most prominently in the southeastern United States. He passionately acted out a childhood memory of his mother urging him to eat, (he works in the film and acting industry and thoroughly enjoyed acting out this scene). In a southern accent, his mother says: "Tony, won't you eat that pie I made," in a sweet, inadvertently (or maybe slyly) guilt-tripping tone. Tony, a deeply empathetic man, only has one response to this, a response which has affected his health considerably.

He tries to make healthy smoothies now to control his diabetes, but regularly gives in to the urges he experiences for sweets and fried foods, which he is far more passionate about. The reason the smoothies aren't working for him is because he is not satisfied on some emotional level. His desire to eat involves much more than just physical hunger and the need to meet caloric requirements. His *why* is plagued by emotions stemming from childhood.

It is beyond the scope of this book to solve a deep-seated problem like Tony's. But as long as we can bring awareness to our needs, we can discover what the causes of our behaviors are. Changing them is a matter of our own will and power to self-heal. The power to heal certainly is within our bodies, not within this book, or in the best doctors. What a good doctor can do is stimulate your own body to heal itself. Perhaps this is why many ancient healers said that God was acting through them to heal the patient; it was never *them* doing the healing. Perhaps the God they referred to was energy from the universe that they managed to tap into.

The point is that it's crucial for you to be honest with your why, especially if it's not just physical hunger. If boredom, pain, or other emotional issues are causing you to eat unnecessarily, you must come to terms with this before applying the methods in this book. The step-by-step methods in the next chapter will *demand* your commitment to self-honesty, so get started *now*.

Beyond what motivates you to eat, you will soon start to tune into how you eat, when you feel hungry, when you get cravings for specific foods, and more. Here are some questions to ponder right now before we get to the methods of *HYMTE*.

- Do you eat because you are hungry? If you answered yes, great. If you answered no, why not?

- Do you stop eating when you are full? If no, why not?

- What motivates you to eat food?

- What makes you hungry?

- What makes you want to eat something in particular?

- When do you get hungry? Why do you think so?

- How do you like to eat? Socializing? Alone? With television? At restaurants? At meetings?

Answer these questions briefly on that sheet of paper. I would refrain from writing down excessively detailed answers. Instead, process the overall feelings and insights you're receiving from your answer, and let them sink into your body. We're going to come back to all of these shortly, in more detail, so these questions are really just a primer.

I've answered these questions myself in my journey to abandoning logic and relying on intuition. I wanted to know if I could really just use my intuition to figure out what to eat. It felt so foreign at first, as I was used to looking up the health benefits of foods *as* I ate them. And I ate them even if I didn't like them.

After I became honest with my *why,* I saw the problem. I was eating for fat loss. It's a lucrative buzzword, and it had me sold from day 1, because I was a chubby kid with man boobs, and I couldn't stand not being physically perfect. I had to let go of these emotions for the time being, gain some fat, and in the process, improve my health. I ignored my natural hunger cues in the obsessive quest to get leaner.

This lack of self-love led to the stifling of my own energies. I was rigid, closed, standoffish, and not jovial much of the time. I see this kind of attitude in a lot of people who become obsessed with achieving leanness and place too much emphasis on appearance, scrutinizing minutiae that no one else notices. People always told me that they didn't notice my man boobs, but I was sure they were wrong because the gyno was clear to me no matter what I wore.

It took me over a couple years to fully embrace eating intuitively. In fact, while writing this book, my own intuitive eating journey improved, because I realized I still occasionally did things based on old ideologies surrounding fat loss, like not eating before working out, or drinking my coffee mostly black.

My *why* is so much different now than in my days of disordered eating. I know that I feel my best mentally and physically when I eat regularly, avoid restricting carbohydrates, and give in to my cravings for sweets. I also have a better understanding of how my body changes. I know that if I start eating too many carbohydrates, my energy does decline. I've become the scientist of my own body, and although I don't have all the answers yet, I'm going a good job in staying energized, and avoiding further health deficiencies caused by a food-centric approach to health. My *why* now is about having energy, feeling happy, and performing at my best. If this means I can't be at 10% body fat anymore, so be it.

Intuitive eating can actually be very difficult for some people, because we've been distrusting our bodies for a long time, and we have attachments to goals such as 'fat loss' which can consume us. Certainly, there are valid approaches to eating that are non-intuitive, but in my opinion, our intuition should validate all scientific approaches to food, exercise, and health. If there's a mismatch, something must be missing, and I think we can sniff it out.

We're about ready to dive into the methods, but before we do, let's set an intention. Say these words to yourself: "I trust that my body, mind, soul, and consciousness has a fascinating ability to keep track of how much food, water, air, and sunlight I need for optimal health. I am ready to wake up my intuition to understand my needs."

7:
How to Eat Intuitively, Step-By-Step

In the pursuit of knowledge,
Every day something is added.
In the practice of the Tao,
Every day something is dropped.
                —LAO TZU (TRANSLATED BY STEPHEN MITCHELL)

I USED TO THINK INTUITIVE eating implied eating *ad libitum*, or eating whatever you want, whenever you want. I've found that this phrasing is perceived as permission to eat junk food all day long. Based on what you've read so far, you may see that this is not intuitive, as your intuition is not going to ever tell you that you crave junk food all day long, unless you've been extremely deprived of food, in which case, it's still not telling you that you need junk food per se, but food in general.

Since the expected outcomes of following an *ad libitum* diet are highly unfavorable, it seems to me that most health writers, health organizations, nutritionists, personal trainers, and the public emphasize the benefits exerting control over appetite. If we don't control it, we may just turn into an Oompa Loompa, right? Wrong. This belief comes from scientific reductionism, devoid of context. Based on these theories, chocolate cake, beer, and pizza are always unhealthy. Believing this, we then aim to eat "healthy" forever—eating clean forever—but occasionally find the need for "balance" by "giving in" to pizza, as if our romantic partner is asexual and we end up cheating on them.

This type of thinking promotes guilt, fear, and anxiety, as well as bingeing, food-obsession, and subclinical eating disorders. It has created a disease. You will say: "Well my partner is asexual but it's still wrong of me to cheat!!" This is the same logic that is used with diet. If your partner is asexual, and sexuality is an important component of your life, your partner cannot satisfy you. If your diet is not satisfying you either, it's not healthy on some level. The fitness industry has come to terms with this with solutions like "flexible dieting" and "cheat" meals. The ketogenic community has come up with "cyclic keto." But there always needs to be some name for the disease of dieting.

The truth is, there is no need to cheat on your diet when you know what your body needs and aren't afraid of giving it to yourself. Our concept of what's healthy and what's unhealthy is going to completely change very, very soon.

Balance is not eating 90% healthy and 10% whatever you want. This thinking is reductionist and inherently flawed. That's not the type of balance you will learn about after finishing this book. That type of balance is black and white. In this view, there are good foods and bad foods. If bad foods, like beer, pizza, and chocolate cake, are *always* bad, why do we crave them? It's because we fucked up.

Your intuition doesn't think chocolate cake is bad. If you're craving it, it means you're getting something out of it. We don't crave snake venom. We don't crave moldy bread. We crave cake, especially when we go on diets that call for extreme restriction, in which case, the cake may be restoring you to a state of balance. But what is balance? Balance is having 50% yin and 50% yang, and 100% whole. Exercise is yang, nourishing foods are yin, and thus, when you crave cake, you're adding yin to balance the excess of yang in your lifestyle. Think of yin and yang as general concepts for now, we won't get too detailed about it.

But what if you eat cake because of your emotions? Well, if you use food to cope with your emotions, there are two scenarios here. One is that you eat cake mindlessly, and after you're done, you're in the same exact state. It's not like your emotions improved at all. In this case, the cake isn't serving you. But on the other hand, your mood improves. In this case, the cake is healthy in a sense.

Whatever the case, it's not bad if food gives you comfort. That actually means it has benefits (intuition is a cognition-independent signal that gives us an awareness of things that increase our comfort, happiness, safety, and survival...remember?). Once you start getting in touch with your intuition you will understand why you're craving that cake (or whatever else it is you crave).

What if cake has processed ingredients? Oh no! "Processed" foods, one of the biggest buzzwords in the health-fanatics mind. **Most food we eat must be processed before consumption.** All that matters as you complete the upcoming steps is that you listen to **what your body tells you.** Don't listen to what anyone else says about how a food impacts your body. Listen to what your body says. Of course, some things take longer to feel, and it's useful to avoid things which most likely post a health risk. But if the particular ingredient you're concerned over is a subject of controversy, chances are the risks were blown up by health fanatics who wanted to be grass-fed, GMO-free, pasture-raised, and organic.

The *HYMTE* approach pays no attention to your beliefs about food; what matters is how your body feels about food, which may completely contradict prevailing theories about it! We will discuss how to make the healthiest choices for our "unhealthy" cravings in chapter 8. Now, I'm all for obtaining food from sources where fewer synthetic ingredients are used, because I have found that I feel better when I do so—I've made that decision after listening to my body.

We've described what intuition is, but how do we apply it to what we eat? It's likely that pre-modern societies and traditions used intuition *and* logic when deciding what to eat. For example, indigenous people in the Andes mountains in Peru would hike long distances to bring kelp to their village for the prevention of goiter. Did this intuitive insight pop out of thin air? I don't know. They used logic too I'm sure, but what matters is that through careful observation and by being the scientists of their bodies and their environment, they found an important solution to their health.

Thus, eating intuitively according to the *HYMTE* approach requires you to be aware of what intuition is, when, where, why, how and for what it calls you, and then implementing the messages it gives you. Yes, you can eat whatever you want. The method to this madness however is figuring out *what* you really want and when you want it.

Intuition is usually a passive process, but by using the steps outlined below we will make it active. Once you get the hang of it, you can operate passively again. But right now, it is going to take some work before you can coast again. Below are the four steps to *HYMTE*:

1. *Develop a palate* by trying different foods.

2. *Evaluate* how you feel afterwards.

3. *Repeat* steps one and two.

4. *Refine*: make sense of the cravings you're getting.

Let's describe each step individually.

STEP ONE: DEVELOP A PALATE

If an infant is raised on formula rather than breast milk, will it crave breast milk? I would guess that an infant never exposed to breast milk would not crave it since no memory of the substance was ever formed. However, since breastfeeding is a universal behavior, maybe infants just know about it somehow. Sucking on a bottle may mimic breastfeeding but whether or not it's perceived exactly the same by the infant is unclear (most likely not).

We are going to assume that without trying a food, you will not have a *memory* of it. So we will disregard the idea that an infant may crave breast milk when it's being fed formula, even though it seems possible to me. Without a memory, your intuition will not be able to tell you if you need it or not. Thus, the first step in following your intuition is *developing a palate* to expand your food memory.

The process of doing this is simple, intuitive, and very natural to most people. All you have to do is try different things and note how you feel about it afterwards. Once you've tried a variety of foods and formed memories of them, your intuition can pick and choose. Without this memory, it cannot.

Now, you don't have to try everything to figure out what works for you. Enough is enough. Imagine for example a Maasai hunter gatherer who already has a diet that keeps him healthy following my advice by deciding to try out the dollar menu at McDonald's one day. He orders a happy meal with a chocolate milk shake (oh boy I sure miss those— not) for breakfast, then for lunch orders authentic ramen in Chinatown, then for dinner eats Swedish meatballs. Good for him.

But I would tell him: "Thank you dear sir. I aspire to be a hunter-gatherer like you, but you aspire to be a confused intuitive eater like me." I am not sure if this type of experimentation will produce better health for an individual whose microbiome is much more diverse than any Westerner's. The Maasai have been eating intuitively; they are connected to what they eat. Perhaps diversifying their diet even more may enrich their lives, but compared to the American, they generally eat more nutritious food and aren't confused about health. We humanoids have been able to live on the Earth perfectly healthfully, much healthier than most modern people in cities live today, without trying foods from across the globe. Not only is it unsustainable to be eating non-locally, it's less fresh.

A conundrum however does arise here which is that in a country like America, people's ethnic backgrounds are from all over the world. Finding an ideal way to eat may thus require some soul-searching. If your background is Italian, try eating authentic Italian food and cooking with the flavors traditionally used throughout the culture.

My experience as an Indian-American is that I strongly prefer my rice with some kind of sauce. Dryer cuisines do not satisfy my palate as much. American food, heavy in fatty, sweet, and salty flavors, don't have the diversity of flavors I crave. Since I've met many non-Indian people who say that Indian food is their favorite type of food to eat, perhaps Indian people are just doing something right with their food that applies to everyone. I do have to say though that some middle-eastern rice and meat is flavored so well with spices that I do not need sauce.

It is beyond the scope of this work to figure out what cuisines from which cultures produce the best health (it's the wrong question to ask anyway, as it can bring out the worst perfectionist in us). One problem in answering this research question is that there are many confounding factors that influence longevity and health and thus suggesting that a diet alone is responsible for the health of a culture ignores all the other equally important aspects of health that we must be aware of. This is very common in the health world I've noticed as people are so disconnected from nature that they attempt to add up the pieces separately when in fact it is all connected.

Lastly, I am not yet certain if consuming a diet that your ancestors ate, if it was a traditional and healthy diet, is always the best for us. I've pondered this when mixing soy sauce, oregano, turmeric, and tomatoes in an Asian-Italian pasta I made once. The product was amazing, but I was hesitant to mix those flavors together initially, since they are used separately in cuisines from different parts of the globe. I told my mom about it and she wasn't excited about it at all.

Our genes are turned on and off based on the things we do, such as foods we consume, and I have a hypothesis that eating the foods that your genes were raised on over the past seven generations may be the best for optimal immune function and health. But this theory doesn't have much research behind it. In fact, it has the potential to be a fad. So when I ate this Asian-Italian-Chinese pasta and noted how great I felt afterwards, I discarded this hypothesis completely.

In step one of eating how you're meant to, you don't have to try *everything* when developing your palate. There is a point where you've tried enough, and it's up to your intuition to determine that. As long as your food memory includes a wide variety of textures, colors, tastes, and other qualities of food, your intuition will have an abundance of options. There is a point where additional diversification will make no improvement in health. You don't need to import superfoods from the Amazon rainforest to maintain health.

Most people do need to diversify their diet. But this idea must be presented with caution, as the chronic dieter sees ideas like this and goes a little crazy. You can use your intuition to figure out when enough is enough and most importantly, take your time with this. We will talk about taking subjective measurements such as how you "feel" after you eat shortly. But before getting to that, let's brainstorm the various *qualities* in food that make them different.

These are qualities that our intuition chooses from when signaling to us what we need to eat. The list below is what came to me intuitively. There is more. And since some of these qualities are subjective, your unique experience with them shapes what they actually are. So feel free to devise your own qualities, on that same sheet of paper you've been using for the exercises thus far (or get a new one). As you read the list below, you may feel into the food. Take your time with that feeling. Enjoy it, savor it, and process it.

FOOD'S QUALITIES:

1. Texture: crunchy (raw bell pepper); soft (brie cheese); hard (nuts); chewy (tapioca); tender (tenderloin steak, tofu); juicy (watermelon); seedy (sesame seeds as a garnish); grainy (bread). Note that most foods usually have multiple flavors and textures.

2. Temperature: hot (soup); cold (refrigerated fruits); frozen; room temperature (fresh coconut water).

3. Color: red (dried chili pepper); orange (bell pepper); green (spinach); spotted (dragonfruit); brown (cooked steak); black (onion seeds, burnt foods); white (cauliflower); purple (cabbage, kale); yellow (squash); blue (blueberries).

4. Smell: aromatic (oregano, thyme); pungent (blue cheese); hot (spicy food); meaty; moldy; flowery (rose). Smell can be very subjective so there are many more possibilities.

5. Taste: sweet (honey, licorice); sour (pickles); salty (soy sauce); pungent (turmeric); bitter (kale); astringent (wine); hot (jalapeno); acrid (burnt food).

6. Constituents: fatty (butter); proteinaceous (chicken, beef); watery (oysters); sugary (watermelon, honey); starchy (rice, potato);

fibrous (vegetables). Note here that there is a distinction between fat and *fatty*. Fat is a noun and isn't a quality of a food. It is a constituent. Fatty is a quality as it describes the food. A food is fatty and a food has fat. For the purposes of eating intuitively, we will stick to the former classification of nutrients (adjectives) as it's more consistent with using our intuition.

7. Production: organic; conventional; grass-fed; wild-caught; 'Round-up ready;' farm-raised; pasture-raised. The quality of soil crops are grown on is also important here. Better soil produces tastier and healthier crops, and we can detect this intuitively.

As you diversify your palate, consider the way the food was produced. Try the same food raised or grown in varying ways. I would recommend sticking to organic produce and meat, grass-fed beef, cage-free and pasture-raised eggs and chickens, and wild-caught fish whenever possible, but use your intuition to guide you.

All of the above qualities may be sensed by our intuition. Macronutrients, non-qualitative aspects of food, may be detected by our intuition as well, and it's why instead of carbohydrates, I listed them as "sugary" or "starchy." Although many people have no idea what foods contain carbohydrates, they can learn to sense how the food satiates them, as a food containing no carbohydrates will satiate them differently than a very starchy food. That's the intuitive paradigm shift I believe can help millions of people reconnect to their food. We don't really need to know what a carbohydrate is to attain optimal health. It might even be better to forget what they are entirely.

You likely won't crave potatoes, rice, and bread all in the same meal. These foods contain mostly carbohydrates, little fat, and little protein. A typical meal reflects what our appetites intuitively seek: a balance of carbohydrates, protein, fat, sugar, fiber, and just as importantly, tastiness. After trying foods that vary in these qualities, you will remember how they make you feel, which is step 2.

Intuition-Building Exercise #6: Food Qualities and Feelings

Before we discuss steps 2-4 of eating intuitively, we are going to develop our ability to sense a food's qualities. You'll need that sheet of paper again, or a new one. For this exercise, pick some of your favorite foods and some of your least favorite foods. Make another 2x2 table like the example ones you'll see below, and title the left column "Qualities" and the right column, "Feelings."

Visualize the food and see which qualities come up in your mind based on the ones we've discussed, or other qualities you've come up with yourself. How do each of the qualities make you feel? Write that down in the adjacent cell of the "Feelings" column to the right. If you can't come up with a feeling right away, leave it blank for now.

In the example below, I pick a food product which I was experimenting with recently: Nutella. I describe Nutella below as sticky, which makes me feel "yucky" if I eat too much. As you can see, "yucky" is a very subjective feeling. Intuition is subjective, abstract, and imprecise at times, while still being wise. So, the feelings you choose to add to your table don't have to be strictly feelings. They can be anything that comes to mind regarding how you feel about the quality of the food. What it *shouldn't* be is a logical understanding of the food, like "sugar." See the example on the following page.

Food: Nutella (was my favorite food for about two weeks)	
Qualities	Feelings
• Sticky	• Yucky if too much eaten
• Sweet	• Yummy, happy, relaxing
• Heavy	• Gross, bleh
• Dry	• Meh, whatevs
• Cooked	• N/A

Recently, I was in love with Nutella. But after two weeks, I noticed signs of inflammation: stiffer joints and throat discomfort/soreness. My feelings predicted this, as they weren't as positive on average as I thought they'd be, and even conflicted with my desire for the addicting taste (there is speculation that vanillin, one of the ingredients in Nutella is addicting). In some ways, Nutella was healthy for me intuitively, and in other ways, my intuition forecasted doom. It was right. I decided not to eat Nutella again after eating three to four tablespoons a day for two weeks. I did experience a reduction in stress and slightly more energy during the days when I ate more sugar however. To maintain that, I will get my sugar fix from less inflammatory foods.

| **Food: Olive** (a food I don't particularly enjoy) ||
Qualities	Feelings
• Smooth	• Comfortable
• Wet and juicy	• Slurp slurp (happy feeling)
• Sour	• Awakening
• Pungent	• Not feelin' it.
• Chewy	• Not rly feelin' it either, bleh.

My feelings if you didn't notice follow a different grammatical code than the writing style I employ throughout the rest of this book. Those immediate feelings that come to me are unadulterated. That's what I love about this exercise. You're working on connecting directly to the feelings food gives you without any filters whatsoever. This is the purest message you're getting, and I believe it is a source of knowledge.

When I wrote above that I wasn't "feelin' it," realize that the words themselves have a specific meaning to *me*. The *words* aren't specific. They just try to capture the feeling, and they can only do so in the context of the experience. So what I mean by "not feelin' it" I am not entirely sure of myself. I just don't like olives a whole lot, and maybe I don't like the chewiness because with each bite I get more of that unique oily and pungent olive flavor. It's an acquired taste.

With this exercise, you may find out that foods you don't really like have some qualities which you actually do appreciate, and foods that you *think* you like have some qualities which aren't so great. If this is the case, you're doing a great job of tapping into your intuitive potential.

For example, you may think that eating peanut butter is unhealthy for whatever reason based on something you read. You may describe it as "aflatoxin" and say that it makes you feel like "cancer." Used as an adjective, "cancer" would be a good description for a strongly negative feeling. But used as a noun, it doesn't fit the bill for this exercise and neither does aflatoxin, as that's not a quality of peanut butter.

Hopefully you've tried the food a few times and are being honest with yourself in this exercise. To double check, try eating the food again and see how you feel about it. If there's mismatch between what you wrote down and what you feel now, create a new 2x2 table for that specific food. This will calibrate your intuition. Since yours may still be developing, this may be an important step to take as you get the hang of receiving and processing intuitive insights.

OK, it's your turn now. Take a deep breath and center yourself before you begin this exercise. Remove distractions. That includes music, cell phones, tablets, and pornography. Jesus, why would that one even be relevant here? I don't know what to expect from people that's why. Just make sure you devote your full attention to this exercise.

Intuition-Building Exercise #7: Food-Focused Meditation

Now that you've had some practice identifying a food's qualities, we will build upon your new skills with a meditation. Don't worry, this exercise is designed to give you a little bit of a break. In the last exercise, the goal was to help you understand the foods you're eating on a qualitative level. This exercise is designed to get you to *feel* deeper into the foods you eat, bringing awareness to any and all sensations, images, and thoughts that arise when focusing on just one particular food. You are welcome to jot down ideas after the meditation, but not during it.

Our feelings can guide us to choose the best things for our lives, just like our intuition can. Intuitive insight can give us a feeling, but feelings and intuition are different things. We don't always get a feeling when we get intuitive insight; this is highly individual. But images, sensations, and random thoughts may arise seemingly out of nowhere from practicing this exercise. Those things are an interaction between you (your unique biochemistry, health, and anything else that plays a role in how food affects your body) and the food.

Think about that. We talk about the health benefits of foods, like say, green bell peppers. I don't know why that just came to mind, but I'm craving watery fruits and vegetables right now. The crunch, the bitterness, and the watery component of it sound appealing to me. I have no idea what this means about my physiology, but I firmly know that a green bell pepper feels far more appealing than a ginger-molasses cookie right now. It's one of the cookies I eat on occasion at a café I frequent, and it's dry, sweet, and concentrated, like Nutella. And with too much of it, I feel "yucky" just as with Nutella.

The health benefits of foods center *solely* around the food. Of course they do. It's not like when you search for the benefits of a food, whatever resource you're using will factor in your unique needs. The implications of this are profound, and this concept extends to everything in the rest of our lives (and it has to do with the holographic universe). This is because the food could not possibly be healthy if we didn't have an appetite for it, and thus it's health benefits depend just as much on us, as the constituents and qualities of the food. It's a two-way street.

Above, when I say "appetite," I refer not only to a physical appetite, but a mental craving for the food, which of course often parallels a physical desire for the food, but not always. If we could digest grass, it would have health benefits. But we cannot digest grass and thus, most of us don't think of it as food (I'm sure there are some freaky people out there who eat grass so that's why I say 'most'). Our realities have a lot to do with how we perceive it. Thus, the way our bodies perceive the food, from sight, smell, taste, and the myriad of processes related to digestion dictate whether or not a food is healthy for us. This concept is very different from the way you may be used to thinking about food.

And, it's just another reason to forego doing research about the health benefits of foods before deciding what to eat, and instead, check in with yourself. The majority of dietary theories that have ever been proposed did not factor in your unique biochemistry, genetics, constitution, and horoscope. This is why I find Dr. Peter D'Adamo's works (Eat Right For Your Type" and "Change Your Genetic Destiny", as well as his other books) so fascinating. He has come up with a method that is designed to factor in your individual interaction with the food. Yet, based on headlines and studies that failed to carry out their aim, many people believe that his approach doesn't work or isn't based on research. It's incredible to see how powerful meaningless headlines influence people's thoughts these days. We are less in tune with our bodies, less aware of it, but inundated and constantly presented with information that cares more about you clicking on it than providing quality information.

In sum, the majority of diets have no personalized element. The *How You're Meant to Eat* approach attempts to make up for this. Although intuitive eating isn't perfect, I know we can discover things that we normally aren't aware of by honing our capacity to feel and tune in to our bodies.

And that's what this exercise is about. On the following page are the instructions.

INSTRUCTIONS FOR EXERCISE #7: FOOD-FOCUSED MEDITATION.

For this exercise, use the same foods you used for the last one, or choose a new group of foods that you like and a group that you don't like. Pick between 3-5 foods for each group.

Now, let all sensations, images, and feelings arise, and without thinking about them, breathe through them. Like regular mediation, the goal here is to reduce mental chatter. If thoughts rise up, be mindful that they are there, but avoid riding any trains of thought. Just experience everything. It's like going on a trip with food; it may be a good trip or a bad trip. Whatever the case, you are connecting to feelings you associate with foods.

You may find that some of these feelings have nothing to do with your intuition. Perhaps you were having the time of your life when you ate your first strawberry and now you love strawberries. Be aware of these types of distinctions. Although this experience with the strawberry may have had a very important role in shaping how the food impacts your health, try to isolate it a little bit—kind of like nutrition science.

You may briefly jot down your experience below each food, but you don't have to. Experiencing it is enough. Figure out what works best for you. This means that you don't have to visualize each food for five minutes as that may not be intuitive nor what benefits you most (don't follow rules!). Once you get the feelings and sensations, you've accomplished the goal for that exercise. It would be interesting to try a couple approaches here.

For example, you could visualize three foods you like first, and experience the positive sensations about them. Of course, like I said, many foods we think we like, we don't intuitively actually like. Then you could visualize foods you don't like, just to focus more on feelings that turn you off from eating something.

Alternatively, you could try switching between foods you like and foods you don't like, going from positive to negative every few minutes or however long you spend in your visualization. Play around with it and have fun! Below is an example table you can construct to jot down a few words associated with the different feelings a food gives you. This is just an example by the way. If you like it, add it to your document. For this type of meditation, it's okay to jot down ideas *while* meditating.

Foods you like

Food:
Feelings:

Food:
Feelings:

Food:
Feelings:

Food:
Feelings:

Food:
Feelings:

Foods You Don't Like

Food:

Feelings:

Food:

Feelings:

Food:

Feelings:

Food:

Feelings:

Food:

Feelings:

STEP TWO: EVALUATE HOW YOU FEEL

Foods contain nutrients which can have infinitely varied effects on us, which we can detect through a plethora of mechanisms involving the gut-brain axis, the gut-brain-microbiome axis, local mechanisms in the stomach like stomach distention (one type of satiety), and communication with adipose tissue. These effects depend as much on the food itself as our unique physiology. Remember, barley grass has different after-effects on a cow than on us. Bread has different after-effects in someone with celiac disease than in someone without it.

Thus, in addition to the fixed physical qualities we discussed in step one, we will also categorize foods based on how they seem to affect us after we ingest them. We will call these *after-effects.* These effects are a mix of qualitative, subjective, objective, and quantitative data. Some are universal to all of us as a species, and others are unique to you and your current activity levels, sleep quality, health, and a myriad of other factors.

There is a large opportunity to find ways to individualize diet. Experiments on intestinal mucosal cells and gluten may answer some questions about how we generally respond to gluten, but there is inherently a degree of variability in scientific research. There is a degree of variability in using your intuition as well (scientists would argue that there is infinitely more variability here as our methods are not quantitative, nor are our settings controlled as if in a laboratory).

One important difference between the two however is that intuition is a mechanism that we all possess and has not changed one bit; whereas, science and research continually evolve. Intuition is thus very reliable once it is awakened, and you can use it to understand how you feel.

Below are examples of after-effects that relate to systems and pathways in the body, that influence your health and physiology. This list is not exhaustive—feel free to devise after-effects suited uniquely to you. But make sure that you can keep sense of them somehow, reliably. The after-effects below pertain to your satiety, metabolism, digestion, mood, and immune system, all of which you may receive feedback about after eating and can track intuitively.

After-Effects of Food:

1. SATISFACTION: THE MOST IMPORTANT

When the food is in your mouth, you should know whether or not it's what you wanted. You might find out instantly, or it might take a few bites. This after-effect is the most important one in the *HYMTE* approach because it's directly related to your craving for the food. As your intuition gets stronger and more calibrated, you will be satisfied by the foods you want. You'll know that the food you're craving is going to taste good. But if it doesn't, you're going to learn why, by adjusting and trying new things. That's step four, refining, which we'll get to shortly.

Being satisfied with what you eat is absent in most discussions on eating healthfully, but I think we all know it's very important. We create "healthy" recipes that seem satisfying but often choose ingredients that on the surface seem healthier (sugar substitutes for example) but isn't what we really want. These superficially healthy foods are designed to trick you into liking something that may boast of having fewer calories or refined carbohydrates (like zucchini noodles which are all the rage right now). Focusing on satisfaction, such a simple concept in my mind, can improve our intimate connection with food, whereas, focusing just on how it's healthy or not healthy is disconnecting us.

How do you measure satisfaction? By feeling it, over the short run and long run. There may be an instantaneous satisfaction, and another one after you've spent some time digesting. One measure of short-term satisfaction is *unputdownability*. When you eat something your body really loves, you won't want to put it down until you've truly had enough of it. When you're eating something you don't really want, it's not going to go down smoothly.

Take alcohol for instance. Some people think they want to drink more alcohol, but this may not be coming from intuition. They drink because they've already had a few drinks and want more. But they aren't tuning in to what they really want. The mind, habits, and addictions are operating here, causing the person to drink much more than they really feel like drinking. Of course, this is a generalization and isn't true in every case.

With food many people might feel like they should eat something because they heard it's healthy. So they continue eating it, but don't really like it that much. According to this book, this is not a sign that the food is what you really want or need. When you operate from intuition, you know that you want the food and this feeling extends far beyond any logical explanation due to the food's estimated health benefits.

Imagine obtaining your caloric requirements from an enteral diet (feeding via a tube). You would receive enough "nutrition" but you wouldn't be using your sense of smell or taste to guide you. In theory (incomplete theories at least), we should be able to obtain all our nutrition requirements from feeding via a tube. We don't "need" our taste buds.

But our taste buds, or gustatory cells, likely evolved to help us survive and determine what foods were good for us, along with our sense of smell. How do you think satisfaction plays a role in your health? What would the consequences of eating unsatisfying food be long term? I'm sure we could adapt to an all-liquid diet, but I'd expect some kind of unknown deficiency to develop long term.

Pay attention to how well the food feeds you. It should be enough. It doesn't have to be unputdownable, but it has to be enough.

2. EFFECT ON SATIETY (FULLNESS)

Some people just aren't aware of when they are satiated, or full. You should eat when you're hungry, and stop when you're full. As you learned in chapter 6, a variety of factors can prevent you from connecting to your intuition, and a common way this affects you is in eating when you're not hungry and not stopping when you're full.

A satiating meal should not have you feeling hungry in another hour. If you're a snacking person who eats multiple small meals a day, you should not feel hungry after fifteen minutes. The purpose of a meal is to replenish and nourish, so you can have energy to move on and do more important things. However, I should say that it's not necessary for optimal health to always eat regular meals. If I'm busy, I will snack and graze.

Satiety depends on what foods you eat, your energy requirements, stress, and possibly hundreds of other factors. After an exercise session for example, you may crave carbohydrates. Eating them will likely satiate you more than eating chicken breasts with lettuce (a meal without carbohydrates).

Satisfaction is related to satiety. If you eat past the point of fullness, or fail to eat enough, you may not be consuming enough truly satisfying foods. Or, you may not be satisfied in general—with life. One patient I observed in medical school was an emotional eater. She was experiencing grief, due to the death of some close friends in recent years. She had put on weight and ate past the point of fullness on a regular basis.

Eating for her became a way to simply drown out the emotions she was experiencing at the time. Not only were the foods she was eating not satisfying, she simply wasn't satisfied in general and had some major health problems, which affected her relationship with food.

There are several types of fullness, and some foods promote certain kinds of fullness better than others. Let's start with a type of fullness that is often promoted as being healthy: stomach distention. Foods that take up more volume in your stomach and therefore may promote greater stomach distention more quickly than calorie-dense foods (like highly processed and refined foods high in sugar and vegetable oils) are often promoted as being healthier alternatives. Not only are they lower in calories, they fill you up faster. Vegetables for instance.

The illusion here however is that this fullness is one-dimensional. There is a difference between being full physically and having the sense that you've eaten enough. That's why if you try to trick your body into thinking you've eaten enough by filling your stomach with these kinds of foods, you will get the sense that you need more food sooner than later. Or, you will compensate somehow by eating massive amounts of peanut butter like I did (half a jar at a time) when I was on the raw vegan diet. My stomach regularly felt distended, but I wasn't as satiated as I am now from eating intuitively.

If I manage to convince myself that I must eat massive amounts of uncooked plant fibers to be healthy, I will experience a second type of fullness too, which is a misnomer really, as it's caused by boredom. In this case, I will stop eating because I am simply bored with chewing. I often experience this with low-palatability foods like raw vegetables, brown rice, and foods which have a low degree of unputdownability, one of the factors that increases satisfaction. I find myself unable to continue eating, seemingly out of boredom, and I know I'll be hungry again in another hour. This is also a one-dimensional type of fullness, in that it's not holistic, and it's not healthy to only aim for this type of fullness. This is the fullness I regularly experienced for *years* by following various restrictive diets. Anytime I've consumed "complex" carbohydrates, like brown rice, in behest of the starchier and saliva-engendering white rice, I felt this kind of fullness. I was neither satiated nor satisfied.

This type of fullness may be beneficial for someone who has consumed weight-promoting foods for many years and is now consequently not only out of touch with their intuition but at an unhealthy weight for their body. The mistake that is often made by those who attempt to be healthy or to lose weight is that they believe that weight-loss promoting foods should be the mainstay in their diet long-term. This is how deficiencies and imbalance can develop.

Let's now consider a holistic type of fullness. This is a signal you get once you've been satisfied and satiated from the foods you ate in your balanced and intuitively-prepared meal. With this type of fullness, you need not feel bloated or as if you've eaten too much, but instead will *know* that you've had enough. There is no pressing desire for any other foods (because you're satisfied). This is ideal.

Mentally note how foods make you full and how they satisfy you overall as you practice step two of eating intuitively. This process will require honesty. Do not give your favorite foods brownie points, no pun intended.

2. EFFECT ON METABOLISM

Is your energy level higher, lower, or about the same after you eat? Maybe you experienced a food coma after all that French toast with maple syrup? Depending also on your own metabolism, the environment, and any other relevant factors, some foods/meals will give you more energy, whereas others may leave you feeling sluggish.

Well what is metabolism? Here I refer to your metabolic rate, or energy levels. Metabolism is defined as the sum of all the chemical reactions occurring in your body. Well, that's a lot of reactions. I don't think we can easily intuit which reactions are taking place when.

What we can understand however is how foods affect our energy levels. The same type of food at a different time of the day than usual, or perhaps on a different day entirely, may produce a different effect on you. There may additionally be a relationship between your cravings and the effect a food has on your metabolism. Slowly piece together the factors other than just the food itself affecting your energy. For example, in the past I did have carb-comas from my pancakes. I added cinnamon and maca powder to them and the problem was solved.

3. EFFECT ON DIGESTION

Digestion involves multiple steps. Problems with digestion can begin in the mouth and can end in the rectum. Are your bowel movements well-formed? Do you have them regularly? If you eat something and you experience bloating, gas, abdominal pain and discomfort, constipation, acid reflux, or other symptoms reflecting poor digestion afterwards, note how you feel after eliminating it.

Here, food combinations will be especially important. We can assess our satisfaction of a single food when it's in our mouth, but it's harder to do the same thing when we eat a meal with a lot of different foods. Trial and error will reveal to you what foods are causing any digestive complaints. If you have a disorder of digestion, make sure to speak with your medical provider about your findings and don't be afraid to use your intuition to figure out what's working and what's not.

4. EFFECT ON MOOD

Do you feel any different emotionally after eating? Do you feel better, or worse? From there, clarify. Happier? Sadder? Bleh? Through the action of neurotransmitters, being satiated, and receiving adequate vitamins and minerals, foods can influence our emotional wellbeing. There are other mechanisms by which food may make you feel better. One of those may be as simple as having enough calories to feel satiated.

Bring awareness to emotions driving you to eat. You may be realizing now that bringing awareness to the various aspects of the self, biology, mind, and digestive tract that govern eating is a central part to eating more intuitively. If you are an emotional eater, use your intuition to decide how your food choices are determined. Are there certain emotions or moods that cause you to eat something?

You may know all of this already. If you're not yet acting on it, then simply knowing it is not enough, is it? You must learn to let go of habits, addictions, and patterns that aren't serving you. Like I said honesty is very important.

As with digestion, combinations of food will have different effects than individual foods. Try to understand this difference through trial and error.

5. EFFECT ON THE IMMUNE SYSTEM

Your immune system monitors antigens on foods. Antigens are proteins that are unique to foods and there is an infinite number of them. When your body recognizes a new antigen, an antibody is made to bind to it. This works great when a pathogen, like *Staphyloccoccus aureus* enters your circulation. It is not so great when antibodies are formed against products from your own glands, like in Hashimoto's thyroiditis, where autoantibodies are formed against the thyroid hormone.

I know that when I drink milk, I have to clear my throat more and my voice is not as resonant. I don't even need intuition here to realize this; it's quite obvious. If you react to foods, stop eating them and see if you react less. Note this, then change your actions and habits. This is the most difficult part of intuitive eating: confronting habits that aren't serving us.

Understanding exactly which after-effect is meditated by the immune system versus digestive system is not important (they may be working together). All that matters is that you are aware of your body.

Keeping Track of After-Effects:

Notice that I am not including any tables in this section. Past a certain point, keeping track of everything is no longer useful. I have no idea if you will use a table here or not. It might look nice, but it might not help you. So I have a better proposition.

Make a specific goal. Through your experiments, if you find that a certain food or meal vastly improves an after-effect you were focused on improving, putting your experiences on paper or on a device may help you remember what it is you're experiencing. All that matters is that you *remember* what's happening and know how to *apply* it to a future experience.

It's too easy to relapse into old ways of living and eating that aren't serving you. Habit creation is hard and I'm just a beginner at this. For example, throughout the process of writing this book, I paid less attention to my intuition with my diet at times. After one week of not listening well to my intuition with diet, I consequently developed a very mild throat discomfort one day. I purchased some pad Thai from a food truck, and it got worse. I was sniffling and became more congested. Thankfully, I didn't get sick, but I knew that I was having some kind of inflammation in my body and perhaps stress from malnourishment and not clearing things out. The mechanisms aren't important. What's important to me is that I knew that I wanted something like *pho,* didn't eat it, then suffered a consequence.

I was craving clearing foods—spicy, aromatic, and soupy foods. I was eating mostly dry foods because they were quicker. When I finally had some pho (a day or two later), I felt much better the next morning. I'm not sure exactly if it was just the pho though. I also had a bag of smelly trash sitting in my apartment that I was waiting to throw out as I filled it up; it might have been smellier than normal, but I didn't notice. All I know is, the next day, I experienced a dramatic difference. I was bubbling with energy in the morning and I realized that I had been living in a fog.

Intuition isn't easy to get precise information from (unless you're highly intuitive) and may not answer all your questions. But what's fascinating is that I was craving a certain type of food, didn't eat it for a while, and experienced ill-health. Once I ate this food, I felt much better. Once I repeat and refine the results, I'll have a better idea as to what could have helped my condition that day. Perhaps I needed the nutrition and anti-inflammatory properties of bone broth. Whatever the case, as I've learned to eat intuitively, I've had experiences like this countless times.

Thus, keeping track of your symptoms is up to you. If you do feel that writing them down or logging them somewhere will help you create habits that improve your qualitative experience of health, I have two suggestions. First, if you work with a healthcare provider, I recommend the app MyMee. It's a program designed to help you keep track of your symptoms and is only available to patients and practitioners (not the general public). A simpler option is to write down your symptoms (being used synonymously with "after-effects"), with the date, and the foods you ate. Keep a chart somewhere, perhaps on Microsoft Excel or on Google Sheets (I prefer the latter for whatever reason but excel has greater functionality). The easiest and laziest option though is to just wing it. Trust your body to tell you what it needs and go from there. That's what I use and what I recommend. It just requires you to follow-up with your insights and be mindful.

As you complete the next two steps of eating intuitively (repeat then refine), you will gain a deeper understanding of what foods affect your health and why. This is an *active* process that requires you to pay attention to symptoms and investigate their solutions through repeated trial and error. It may sound tedious, but that's part of taking control of your health and being the scientist of your own body.

Whether you choose to record your after-effects or not, remember that what matters is progress. It matters that you *remember* notable symptoms and changes due to diet. And it matters that you can rely on your experiences to inform future food choices.

If you experience a lot of health problems currently and react to food, I recommend keeping a detailed record of symptoms. It could look something like what is illustrated in the table below. If your goals are simply to have more energy and connect to your food, you can practice bringing awareness to your unique after-effects with food. Trust your body to tell you what's going on.

Example Table to Track After-Effects of Food and Symptoms				
	Duration (days, weeks, or months)	Severity (1-10)	Progress (0-100%)	Things that make it better
Irritability	10 years	10	5%	Sex and nature walks

In addition to this table, make another table for each symptom you're trying to improve. For example, if your throat gets congested and you have to clear it from eating certain foods, add a table like the one below. In this below table you can add any lifestyle variable that is causing a symptom you notice.

Throat congestion			
	Eliminating Milk	Sushi consumption	Stress
Progress (0-10)	10	2 (sushi makes my throat congested, depending on the quality)	2 (makes it worse)
Duration of effect (minutes, hours, days, etc.)	48 hours (it takes 2 full days for my throat to clear up after eliminating milk, that's how long some allergens take to go away)	2-3 hours	1 hour

Set a time to add to your tables to track your progress. Either make a quick update right after your meals or do it all at the end of the day. Whichever method you choose, as you learn to connect what, how, why, when, and where you eat with the after-effects you get with food, you will connect with it on a deeper level and be more informed about what's working for you.

Intuition-Building Exercise #8: Eating Slow & Silently

I mentioned earlier how distractions can prevent our intuition from working properly. So, for this exercise, you are instructed to eat without any distractions at your table, or wherever it is that you eat. In addition, you are instructed to bring awareness to each morsel of food you touch with your mouth. If you're like me, you like to shove food down your throat when you're hungry. If you're not, great—you can still practice eating mindfully and more slowly.

If you like to scroll through media on your phone while you eat, put it away—far away. Make sure you would have to get up in order to get it just as an extra precaution. If you always eat socially, forego that for the time being—no talking here. It's just you and your meal. If you like to watch TV or stream TV shows on Netflix while you eat, put that away too. Make sure the remote is nowhere in sight. Turn your computer off. Dirty your hands with food so you are less tempted to distract yourself.

Everyone is different here and has different degrees of difficulty with turning off distractions. They are addicting, and thus extra discipline is required to practice exercises like this. I actually love watching something entertaining while I eat. But nowadays I also like to evaluate what I'm eating to better understand my meal and my food.

As I develop my cooking skills, I can use my senses to evaluate my product. How does it go down? How unputdownable is it? Do the tastes complement each other? How do I feel about it? These are the types of questions you should ask yourself as you practice this exercise. But to answer these questions, do not write anything down. Focus on the feelings and experiences that come up as you focus on each bit. With time, you can certainly eat with television or other distractions and still know when to stop eating.

With regard to the mindfulness component of this exercise, your first obstacle may be distracting thoughts. When thoughts arise, because they will, bring awareness to the existence of the thought, without thinking about the thought. Avoid riding the train of thoughts that arise, and instead bring your attention back to what you're eating. Most importantly, never give up on this. Meditation takes time and most people make excuses about the amount of time they have in a day. It does take 20-30 minutes out of your day to meditate and it will take time to practice the exercises in this book. But the purpose of exercise is to strengthen, so putting in the time is worth it if that's your goal. Make sure you have a goal of yours in mind as you perform these exercises.

The instructions for this exercise are simple. Remove distractions and focus on the after-effects and qualities of what you're eating as you eat it. *Chew your food more slowly and more thoroughly as well.* This will increase your interaction with that food. But long term, you may intuit that you don't need to chew each bite of food ninety-nine times as per that ancient Chinese saying you may have come across.

And don't forget, satisfaction is the most important after-effect in the *HYMTE* approach. You may be satisfied on some levels with what you eat but not on others. The Nutella I was eating for example satisfied my taste cravings to an extent, but started to bother my throat eventually, and therefore, became unsatisfying overall. Things may change, and we'll discuss how to deal with this shortly.

The more you practice the exercise, the more calibrated you will become to your needs. In chapter 9, I will provide recommendations for how often you should practice this exercise, along with the others. For now, get the hang of it. Compare how the foods make you feel when you're fully present with it versus when you have distractions at your side.

Step Three: REPEAT!

You now have a richer memory about what foods you like and what you don't like and are able to correlate it with after-effects. These memories include how foods make you feel mentally, how they make your GI tract feel, how well you digest them, the quality of your bowel movements, the quality of your sleep, and a myriad of other factors.

This step in the intuitive eating process requires you to rely on that memory, without thinking about it. Here's how it's going to work:

- You will get hungry.

- You will wonder what to eat. Here's where intuitive insight will come to you. Let it do so.

- **Eat** what you intuitively want to eat.

- **Evaluate** how you feel.

- **Adjust** and **refine**.

- **Repeat**.

As I mentioned earlier, using intuition can be uncomfortable because a lot of the knowledge doesn't seem certain to the logical mind, which many of us are accustomed to relying on for decision-making. If this feels slightly uncomfortable and uncertain, *you're on the right track*.

Repetition however is a necessary step in the scientific method. We must repeat our experiments and have others repeat the same experiment, and get similar results, to confidently draw a conclusion. Repetition of your trials will reveal to you a pattern. The overall pattern here is to learn to detect intuitive insight, listen to it, follow it, and repeat it, until you understand your body on a deeper level.

STEP FOUR: REFINE

The fourth step to the *HYMTE* approach is to refine your methods. Since this is first and foremost a guide, it truly is designed to help you understand how to figure out what you need. That means it may be confusing. I know I sound like a broken record at times, but once again, it took me a few *years* to abandon the disconnected logical thinking I relied on to guide food decisions and fully embrace intuition.

If you are starting to choose foods more intuitively and now have more energy, clarity, and a greater subjective sense of well-being, I'm proud of you. You are learning about what your body wants and connecting to it. Instead of eating mindlessly, you eat mindfully.

But perhaps you have some questions or are a little confused about how to go about following your intuition. Remember that the goal is to optimize the *after-effects* of eating. Specify which after-effects are most relevant to you. Recall, these after-effects include the way food affects your digestion, metabolism, cognition, and emotions, as well as any other after-effects you find suitable. For example, beyond satiating your appetite, you could monitor how well eating a food satiates your soul. Is what you're eating "soul food?" Or, if you want to experience more energy after you eat, that should be your focus.

On a molecular level, after-effects include the effect foods have on your cells. Chlorogenic acid for example, present in the coffee I'm drinking right now, is mildly anti-diabetic. This objectifiable after-effect is not the kind we will rely on to eat intuitively. It's just an example of why after-effects are important. In fact, the healthiness of food is determined (by conventional nutrition science) entirely by its after-effects.

The good after-effects are what you want, and refining your intuitive insights to optimize them is most likely important to you. For others however, feeling satisfied with having a basic framework for choosing what to eat, with less confusion and more clarity, is enough. But many health-conscious people do deeply care about having healthy levels of certain biomarkers, hormones, and other things that influence our health quantitatively, and like to get into the nitty-gritty.

With the methods in this book, you can still do all that while eating intuitively. Say for example you crave Nutella, like me. You eat it, and observe how it makes you feel. You repeat the process. To *refine* this, try something similar—something with similar qualities. It doesn't even have to be a "healthier" version of Nutella. Perhaps it's something else your body wants when it craves the soft, spreadable, chocolate, sugary-spread that is Nutella.

I tried this the other day. I purchased a 'healthier' version of Nutella, and it simply didn't taste as good. I also ate more of it than the Nutella because the original spread is much tastier and I wanted the sweet taste. Oh well. I'm taking a break from Nutella for a little while though now. I'm on a pho kick. This is what I call refining the process. It's about understanding the craving and trying other versions of whatever food you're craving or foods with similar qualities, to better pinpoint your needs.

Make sure to continue tuning into your body and asking yourself what it is that you want. Going for a walking meditation in nature may help. I would suggest using the list of qualities earlier in this chapter to identify which ones you are looking for as you advance in your intuitive eating journey.

Use what you've learned from steps 1-3 to start substituting foods with each other to see if they give you the same beneficial qualitative after-effects which you can perceive with your intuition. Repeat as usual, and refine further, until you find something that works for you or has a desired effect. Making sense of your intuitive cravings will be discussed further in the next chapter.

In conclusion, refining involves substituting foods that you enjoy with other foods that have similar qualities, and observing how you feel afterwards. This expands your food memory and will help you make clearer food choices in the future.

It is now time to take everything we've just discussed and put it into practice.

Intuition-Building Exercise #9: Grocery Bonanza

This is your final exercise. It involves taking all the principles in this book and applying it to your typical shopping experience with food. You can perform this at a grocery store, farmer's market, butcher shop, or anywhere else you get food, including directly from your garden or even a hunt of sorts. For the purpose of this exercise though, we will choose a grocery store as it's the most common food-shopping experience. However, there isn't as much diversity of food as we'd think at a grocery store. The ideal place to perform this exercise would be at food markets, like farmer's markets, fish markets, and places where food is very fresh. Start with a grocery store if that is where you typically do your shopping, and then do this at a food market of sorts.

The purpose of this exercise is to build upon your understanding of why you like the foods that you like, and don't like the foods that you don't like. You're going to be walking through a grocery store practicing bringing up the sensations, feelings, and thoughts you get when you see a food in front of you. In previous exercises, we brought up the food in your mind (unless you had it with you during the exercise).

You're going to need to be very hungry for this exercise. Make sure you haven't eaten in several hours and perhaps even plan a workout before this experience. You don't have to water fast for three days before this exercise, but you are welcome to. I need you to be salivating for this.

Don't make any lists before going to the store. You will get what you need, but we are going to shop a bit differently. Here are the steps:

Instructions for Intuition-Building Exercise #8: Grocery Bonanza

1. Walk through each aisle of the grocery store. Start with one side of the store, and make your way to the other side, going through **each aisle.** Feel free to add items to your basket or cart as you do this exercise, but make sure to go through every single aisle. If you'd prefer just to focus on the exercise, do not bring a cart or basket with you. I know you'll be very hungry but just hold off from opening that jar of Nutella in the store.

2. In each section of the store **let your eyes land on the foods they like**. Intuition once again is a signal that comes to you. The things you are drawn to will pop out at you. As you find foods you like, start to embrace the feeling they give you. Understand why you want this food. Visualize, as you have done in previous exercises. For example, I love pears. I like the sweet and juicy quality of pears. I prefer them over most apples.

3. After you've practiced this exercise with a food that you were naturally drawn to, focus on a food that you're not drawn to. The apples for example might be a bit too tart. I don't like that. But the apples I find at farmer's markets are far better tasting.

4. Find a few foods in each aisle to repeat this process with. Pick a few foods you like, and then experience the sensations of foods you don't quite like that are in the same aisle. This exercise will take you at least a half-hour to complete.

As you perform this exercise, you will learn to understand what separates foods you like from foods you don't like. You may also understand why you don't like certain foods, now that you understand foods' qualities better. Maybe there were foods you thought you didn't like because you read they were "fattening" but now can appreciate certain qualities about them and can find a place for them in your diet if your intuition approves.

This is an exercise you should repeat when you're in a grocery store again. In your future visits, you don't have to go through each aisle, but can practice in the sections of the store that you need to obtain your groceries from. It's an exercise that can help you remove biases and prejudices about a food based on your beliefs, and connect to it on a deeper level. It's also an exercise you can practice to compare your sensations in different food-containing environments. For example, you can compare the sensations you get about the foods you're drawn to at a farmer's market vs. a grocery store. Your intuition will probably appreciate qualities about foods that seem fresher over foods that don't look as fresh at a grocery store. But let's be thankful for grocery stores, eh?

Or say you go to a wine tasting event. You can use your intuition not only to sniff out your next hot future date, but the differences in the wine. Maybe you can't discern too much at first, but with time, you'll get better at recognizing what you like and don't like about a food. Once you've completed this exercise, congratulate yourself. Being able to choose foods based on purely your instinctual desire for them is a major accomplishment. You are now able to eat how you're meant to.

8:
Understanding Your Cravings

YOUR INTUITION DOESN'T KNOW why you like what you like. It picks something that enhances your comfort and survival. Considering the obvious fact that the majority of foods we have available to us at grocery stores is of suboptimal quality and nutrient density, it is vitally important that we attempt to understand what our intuitive cravings mean for optimal health. Going extreme in any direction, whether it be logical eating, or intuitive eating, is not going to produce the best results.

For example, imagine that one day you get hungry and crave a burger from a fast-food chain. According to much of what's said in this book, you should totally eat it. But what about next time? That's where step four, refining, comes in. We need to try *new* things to figure out what matches the intuitive desire the best.

In the case of the fast-food burger craving, the way I recommend breaking down the craving is by first performing food-focused meditation and listing the food's qualities, as we did in exercises 6 and 7. I suggest doing the food meditation first, because that exercise is about tuning in. Exercise 6 involved writing down qualities of foods, which is a more active exercise. I want you to in these situations learn to go by feel. Sniff it out.

Yes, I know it might seem weird if you stand outside that fast-food restaurant, close your eyes, and look like you're on an acid trip. You can hide somewhere and practice the meditation if you're afraid of looking odd. The goal is simply to connect to your feelings and sensations, which many of us have ignored and which isn't a common part of our discussions in nutrition. This will clarify your desire for the food.

Now if you decide that there are qualities of this food that you do like, you should eat the food. Then, as soon as it's in your mouth, you will begin to calibrate. You will see whether or not your intuitive insight about this food matches your satisfaction to the food. Remember, satisfaction is the most important. Maybe you need those fast carbs in the bread. Or maybe you just want the meat and not the bread. Whatever the case, you will figure this out by touching base with your satisfaction level. How does the bread feel as you chew it and mix it with your saliva with everything else in that burger? What about the lettuce? Do you hate lettuce? If so, modify this burger to your liking at home and experiment with it. By doing this, you go through the four steps we discussed in the last chapter.

Don't worry, it's not the end of the world if you eat some genetically-modified food or refined white sugar. Maybe you read somewhere that it makes your brain look like that of a cocaine addict. There was a terribly clickbaity article that as usual misrepresented the research and suggested that eating white sugar is as addictive as cocaine. People got scared. Pay no attention to those headlines that are popping up in your mind. As the scientist of your body, your job is to validate that research with your own personal n-of-1 experiments.

I think many of us have this hope that if we only ate high quality, local, and fresh foods, we would not crave sugary foods or other junk foods. But perhaps home-made foods containing some sugar can actually improve our health and metabolism. I remember years ago, when I was not eating properly while training like an athlete, I craved skittles candy really badly (I loved those as a kid). I realized that I wanted some sugar. After long workouts, I occasionally find myself eyeing it at the grocery store during checkout. What I've learned about this craving is that it means I need food ASAP. Since skittles are a fast way to obtain a lot of sugar, which lowers stress, my body sees it as an attractive option.

When I used to eat "clean" (it's a term that the fitness industry came up with to focus on losing fat) I noticed that despite what seemed like a complete meal, consisting of some low-glycemic starchy vegetables, other vegetables, spices, and meats, I was *still* craving sugar. When I learned to eat sugar, I finally felt satisfied. Dessert is a universal thing, I realized. After Indian lunch buffets, there is always a dessert. The sweet helps to balance out the spice from the main dishes. Maybe dessert is an essential part of a healthy diet. What!? I know. We've been lied to.

Below I've listed several areas where you may have questions about applying the methods in this book. It will provide guidance on making sense of the cravings you get, especially if optimal health is your goal.

Foods vs. Meals

We don't eat one food at a time unless we're snacking. We typically eat a few foods at a time in a single meal. In a single bite, we may mix more than one food together, flavored with multiple ingredients. Yet, we've still focused on individual foods a lot throughout this book. This is not a problem. You can judge your liking and appetite for each food, flavor, texture, etc., both individually and together with other foods.

Synergy happens when you eat multiple foods. Thus it makes sense to evaluate the combined effect of foods together. Nutrition science isn't very good at doing this, but you do it all the time. Bring your attention to the after-effects of individual foods as well as the synergistic effects of eating them together. You don't have to try too hard. The intuitive insight will come to you. You have to trust your body.

Going back to the fast-food burger, when the different qualities of different foods are together in your mouth at the same time, you can certainly understand which ones appeal to you the most. You will become a burger connoisseur if you keep up a practice like this. Call it your burger yoga practice if you will. Breathe through each bite, and be mindful.

Once you get the hang of identifying a food's qualities, start identifying which qualities mix together well in your meals. Thankfully, the wheel won't be reinvented. There's an intuitive process to preparing a delicious meal with complementary tastes and textures and once you start paying attention, you'll know how to construct healthy meals not based on the ingredients or health benefits, but how they make you feel balanced.

Overall After-Effects, and Individual After-Effects:

There are many ways we can reduce health to its parts. We can also reduce food cravings to its parts. But remember that there is always a whole. You may be craving one food in particular, but it's a sign of something bigger—some single need. And after you eat well, you have a singular general sense of satisfaction.

We discussed a variety of after-effects in step two, but I did not elaborate on their interconnectedness. When experience good health, your heart, lungs, brain, muscles, and digestive organs function in harmony together, like a prosperous civilization. Consider the prosperity of your body after it is fed, by bringing awareness to a *general* sense of health and wellbeing as correlated with the foods you are intuitively consuming, rather than just specific after-effects.

Knowing When You Are Full

Those with a history of eating disorders often have trouble understanding when they're full. Those with a history of dieting for fitness competitions and tracking their calories and macronutrients may also struggle with understanding fullness. These people may need to eat much more than they realize to truly feel satisfied, as long-term dieting makes one ravenous.

If this is you, trust that with time you'll learn how to follow your hunger cravings. Set an intention do so. Stop restricting, that's very important. If you learn to let go of limiting beliefs, guilt, and fear surrounding what to eat, *and* apply the *HYMTE* approach, you will learn to go with those foods that call to you at any given moment. Avoid the temptation to track your calories and macronutrients. You shouldn't ever have to do this for optimal health! Tracking seems like a great idea to lose weight and it may be, but it's not a tool for achieving optimal health in my opinion.

Beyond chronic dieters, many people don't know when they are full simply because *they are not listening*. Thus, you want to bring your attention within. This will get the process started. For me personally, I get full when I am "bored." We move on from things when we've had our fill. It is not productive for us to continue. That's what feeling full is like for me. My stomach may have more room, but my body has energy and I want to move on and do something else. Find out what drives you to *stop* eating.

"Chemicals"

The increasingly health-conscious consumer is aware that foods should not contain many chemicals, which has a slightly metaphorical definition, and describes synthetic chemicals added to foods, like preservatives, food coloring agents, artificial sweeteners and flavorings, and other additives only, and not all chemicals such as those our cells run on. Those who fear "chemicals" may find themselves at a crossroad when their intuition asks for a certain food but their beliefs about chemicals call to stay away from that food.

Eat it. Just eat it. Follow your body, and go through the four steps as I said before. Maybe your beliefs are wrong. There are some chemicals in foods that might be best to stay away from. But try it once, and let your intuition tell you if the food is safe. It will have the right answers. I personally stay away from foods with a lot of chemicals as they don't taste good and I get a bad feeling about them.

Things Change

The same food, at the same time, may not give you the same subjective after-effects each time. It's important to realize that your body's needs change. If you become attached to your ideas of how the food affects you, you will be disappointed when things change. Accept that this will happen, and you won't be disappointed. Be able to adapt to new information and you will feel emotionally more resilient in light of new changes.

There Is No Perfect

Intuitive eating is not an exercise in perfectionism. If you eat something that perhaps wasn't the best for you at a given moment, first, forgive yourself, and second, realize that your body adapts to things and it isn't the end of the world. Refine and calibrate your intuition by trying it out substitutes.

As a previously perfectionistic eater, I realized that my ambitious personality led to eating in a way that was deteriorating my health. I thought my diet was perfect, yet I was not performing at my peak, physically or mentally. Since those times, I've realized that perfectionism is in general a bad idea with food. Perfectionism can also lead to disordered eating habits in the long run. For mental peace and happiness with food, we must learn to let go of what our minds may have to say about a food, and let our bodies tell us instead. If I hadn't been a perfectionist, I wouldn't have written this book.

9:
One-Month Timelines

BELOW IS A SUGGESTED TIMELINE for practicing the various exercises presented in this book until you get to a point where eating intuitively feels automatic. Sometimes I forget what it was like to think excessively about what I ate, because now I sometimes don't think enough. Finding a balance between planning meals based on nutrition facts and validating those facts with subjective experience takes time and attention.

The exercises I've presented in this book are all designed to connect you to your food and enhance your intuition. But if you only practice them once, you may not get to the place you want to with your intuitive eating habits. So here is a suggested one-month timeline for practicing the methods in this book, along with the exercises, after you've already completed them once while reading this book.

I've separated these timelines into two groups. The first group is for those who are recovering from an eating disorder, have a history of chronic dieting, and are confused about what to eat. This group is ideal for anyone who has ever believed strongly in one dietary ideology before and/or has studied nutrition. The second group is the layman; people who feel confused and overwhelmed by the amount of conflicting information on what to eat but haven't had a past of disordered eating or obsessive nutrition researching tendencies. This is ideal for someone with a general interest in being healthy.

Condition #1: Confused And/Or Recovering from an Eating Disorder

If you currently are an overthinker and are recovering from an eating disorder, my suggested plan for you is a bit more intense. You need to confront the thought patterns that have dictated your life for a while now and heal.

WEEK 1

For **one meal per day**, have a piece of paper with you at your kitchen table, or wherever it is that you eat. On this piece of paper, practice the food qualities and feelings exercise (exercise #6, p. 122) *as you eat*. In this exercise, we described the qualities of foods and how those qualities made us feel. As you experience each bite, write these things down. Now, you can also write down the qualities/feelings for a combination of foods, based on what's on your plate. Eggs with salt for instance could be one combination. It doesn't have to just be about a specific food.

After you eat, check in with your feelings about the foods you ate, as in exercise #4 (p. 97). As you get better at listening to your body, your beliefs surrounding what foods you should eat will change. Recall that in this exercise we picked individual foods and wrote down overall feelings and thoughts that arose about this food. Do this to check in with your meal after you've finished eating it. And once again, the point of *HYMTE* is to connect to food. I suggest practicing this exercise for just one meal per day for a week to enhance that connection, but I would recommend for the rest of the day to simply enjoy what you're eating.

Next, practice distraction-free eating as much as possible this week. I suggest eating mindfully as described in exercise #8 (p. 145) for at least two meals a day. During the other meal(s), relax and let yourself eat socially, with TV, or with your phone. You may find that you actually prefer eating without distractions once you get used to it because it can provide a new source of pleasure that we often ignore from rushing through our meals.

By the end of the week, redo exercise #5 (p.107) to check in with the factors potentially blocking your intuition. How have your beliefs changed? How much are you still thinking about food? What progress have you made here?

Further, each night this week, practice exercise #7 (p. 126) where you meditate on a variety of foods and bring up the thoughts, feelings, and sensations that arise. Do this with the foods you ate that day to check in with your intuition, or pick the same foods you chose when you first did the exercise—it's not very important which ones you pick.

In the same vein, practice a modification of exercise #3 (p. 77), the focused meditation exercise, where you picked an emotionally-charged recent event and picked up on intuitive insights about that situation, daily. Perform it again exactly as described, or alternatively, practice it with events throughout the day. This can include the random people you see, current events, and any other event during your day. Practice being aware of the immediate judgments and intuitive insights that arise from these situations.

Lastly, take one day out of your week to spend an hour in nature somewhere, as in our first exercise (p. 6). The goal here is to perform these exercises regularly throughout the week to allow your intuitive capabilities to grow.

WEEK 2

This week, intuitive eating should become a little more passive. It may still be very confusing, but at least you know how to view food from a different lens and can identify its qualities. If your thinking and beliefs around food have reduced in intensity, you are now permitted to eat socially, with TV, and other distractions if you so choose, as long as you are able to tell when you're full and when you're hungry. I recommend at least one meal of the day be spent eating mindfully in silence.

Add new foods to your palate each week, evaluate them, repeat, refine, and only then come to a conclusion about how healthy it *feels* for your body. Continue practicing the food-focused meditation exercise, or exercise #7 (p. 126), each night. At the end of the week, redo exercise 5 (p. 107) once again to check in with factors blocking your intuition. Ask yourself how your beliefs have changed like I described in week 1.

WEEK 3

Same as week 2.

WEEK 4

Before deciding what exercises to perform this week we will tune in to see what kind of progress we've made. For the confused dieter or the individual recovering from an eating disorder, there are a few areas where we need to tune in to before deciding how we will move forward: thinking, clarity, intuitive ease, and separately, body image.

Thinking

Are you still overthinking what you will eat? Are you analyzing every health problem you're having? Are thoughts of vitamins and minerals in food still dominating your ideas on what foods are healthy or not?

If this is the case, don't worry, as these things take time. Here's the plan. Remove the factors causing you to think. Remove the stimuli that got you here. This includes calorie trackers and all sources of information regarding the logical aspects of eating. Remove them and immerse yourself in the less-predictable world of abstract intuitive living. Go back and practice exercise #1 (p. 6), where you walked and meditated in nature. But instead of an hour, spend all day in nature; it rejuvenates.

Next, look at that sheet of paper from week 1 where you wrote down the feelings you got from food, in the food-feelings exercise. If you're an overthinker, you will have feelings about foods that reflect whatever negative things you've read about them from wherever you get your information. For example, you may think that fried foods are "unhealthy." Your challenge here is the following: make a list of seven "unhealthy" foods that you're still somewhat okay with eating and write down what feelings you associate with these foods. Then, over the course of this week, eat each one of those foods.

If I were instructing the 2013 version of myself to perform this exercise, I would recommend for him to start with eating these seven foods: a soda, a burger from a fast-food restaurant, toast with white bread, skittles candy, a 10" pizza, a good quality beer, and a donut. If I had done this in 2013, I would have experienced the after-effects of each of these foods, and realized that they weren't too bad. I've tried all of these foods since that date except for the skittles, as my intuition tells me to stay away from the food colorings and the other ingredients in those types of candies. As far as the burger, I haven't been to McDonald's, but I've found a few restaurants that were acceptable.

Clarity

Are you able to make clear choices about what you want to eat? Or are you stopping yourself, perhaps because of beliefs, distractions, or any of the other intuition-blocking factors? Remember that intuition is fast. You receive insight and make decisions quickly once you're in tune with your intuition. Therefore clear choices are quick choices.

If you're struggling with this, my suggestion is to first figure out what's stopping you. Is it guilt? Fear? Beliefs still? Go back to exercise #5 (p. 107), where you identified the factors blocking your intuition. Be honest with yourself about this, and dig deeper into any of the factors you listed when you first performed this exercise. For example, say you're experiencing some guilt deep down somewhere. Meditate on this feeling, as we did in our focused meditation in exercise #3 (p. 77), and see what comes up. Perhaps you'll find insight as to where this feeling is coming from. Introspection will reveal answers to you. Write down the results of your focused meditation and hopefully this will clarify your decisions.

Intuitive Ease

Once you get the hang of eating intuitively, it's easy. You know when, why, how, and what to eat (or even who—it's a metaphor okay, relax). But if it's not easy yet, the problem may lie in your understanding of a food's qualities. My recommendation is to expand upon exercise #6 (p. 122), where you identified qualities of foods, and now add several more foods to your list in this exercise. Remember that the first step of the *HYMTE* approach involves diversifying your palate. In order to do this, you need to try a lot of new foods.

Try this exercise with foods you haven't tried in a while or have never tried before. As you eat the food, or even beforehand, notice the qualities, like the color, texture, shape, taste, etc. Write down how you feel about that quality, as in, how you feel about eating a food with that quality. Maybe it resembles other foods you've had, or maybe it provides your appetite with something slightly new entirely. If your diet hasn't been varied lately, something in your body will awaken when you diversify the qualities of foods in your diet.

Throughout the week, either after meals or before bedtime, practice exercise #7 (p. 126), the food-focused meditation. Imagine these new foods you've added to your diet and just experience the thoughts, sensations, and ideas that arise. Hopefully they're positive.

Repeating exercises 6-8 will hopefully improve your ability to "sniff" out what you need and follow your intuition. This will over time lead to clearer and easier decision-making regarding what's going into your body.

Body Image

People who aren't confident or happy about the appearance of their body often eat non-intuitively, because their focus is on changing the body. If a body image problem is preventing you from eating intuitively, acknowledge it as an intuition-blocking factor. Decide if you're willing to make a compromise on this right now for the sake of your health, or if you prefer to continue pursuing an aesthetic goal. If you do decide to put off the aesthetic goal and instead, focus your efforts on connecting to food, you may be surprised to see that when you follow the steps of *HYMTE*, you aren't going to turn into Humpty-Dumpty.

I have a faith that our intuition wants to guide us to a happy place. Thus, when you learn to be honest about what foods make you feel good, you'll likely choose foods that also keep you at a healthy body weight. *HYMTE* isn't a weight loss book, or a book about gaining weight. It's about connecting to nature, which means, either scenarios could come true depending on where you are. And of course, if your goal is to get six-pack abs, you may have to eat non-intuitively to get there, depending on your genetics and response to exercise.

Personally, I find more beauty in the intricate complexity of nature and connecting to intuition than I do in six-pack abs. The latter is superficial, and although interesting to an extent, being in tune with nature has broader implications for our health and is certainly my personal health goal.

Make a decision now about what you're doing to do with your body image issue. If you do decide you want to experience more connection, practice the nature walk again (exercise #1) and the time travel exercise (p. 61) as these two can help you reset mentally. Then, tune in with which exercises you think will benefit you the most, and practice those this week. Also see which of the above three areas, (intuitive ease, clarity, and thinking), need the most adjustment and follow the suggested plan there.

NOW THAT YOU'VE TUNED IN...

The rest of my suggestions for week 4 centers around the contents of chapter 8 and in step 4 of *HYMTE:* refining. This step involves replacing the foods you've evaluated the after-effects of, and repeating the process. How do similar foods make you feel? Say for example you craved a Twinkie. You felt okay eating it, but suspect, intuitively of course, that there are other trans-fat-free options which could satisfy you just as much (most likely you weren't even satisfied eating it).

By trying out Twinkie substitutes, you go through steps 1-4 again. Your intuition is getting calibrated. I went through this process with Nutella. I decided that the substitutes just didn't cut it, and decided that I needed to cut Nutella from my life because it was inflammatory. I have had intermittent desires for it, but as long as I eat a balanced diet with some sugar, I do fine without it.

Now, as the scientist of your own body, you can come up with your own innovative solutions. You've tried all the exercises now, perhaps more than a few times. Figure out what works for you, what doesn't, and innovate. I want you to build upon all the progress you've made and do it even better, making it as personalized as possible. Nature doesn't follow script, as far as I know.

Condition #2: Generally Confused and Wants to Know How to Eat

If you don't have a past of disordered eating, but just feel confused by all the information out there, the suggested one-month plan is to enhance your intuition and develop self-trust. I recommend carrying a journal to write down your sensations.

WEEK 1

With each meal, snack, or drink of water, coffee, tea, or alcohol this week, your task is to tune into how well you are satisfied. Satisfaction involves short term validation, which takes place as your meal makes contact with the first part of your GI tract, your mouth. Satisfaction also involves how well your body digests food. Practice exercise 9, "Grocery Bonanza" (p. 150) four times this month. You can do it once a week, when you shop for groceries.

If you notice anything strange about after-effects or your cravings, write that down in a separate food journal. Create a spreadsheet too if you'd like, and pay attention to what parts of your health and body seem affected when you eat different things. Go through the list of after-effects listed in chapter 7 and pay attention to which systems are better or worse with different foods and combinations of foods.

You may feel at times like this is too much for you to do yourself. But it's not. You must believe in yourself. No one can do this as well as you can. This is what intuitive eating is about, and we've done it for millions of years.

WEEK 2

At the end of the last day of week 1, decide how well you're doing. Is this starting to make sense? What areas need more work? Beliefs? Emotions? Still experiencing a lack of connection to intuition? If the idea of intuition is totally unfamiliar to you, it will take much more than a week to get the hang of it. Have faith and make the best progress you can, but realize it will take more time to completely flow with intuition in your life.

If you decide that you need to work on getting in tune with your natural hunger cues, focus on what takes place before you get hungry. Are there any particular events that precede the desire to eat? Or does it happen like clockwork? Read through chapter 6 again and write or type out your answers to the questions posed.

If you feel that you don't understand intuition, practice exercise 1 and 2 again, on the first and second day of this week respectively, or on the first day if you can. Exercise #1 (p. 6) was the walking meditation in nature. Spend as much time as you can afford in a natural environment without distractions. Exercise #2 (p. 61) was our time travel exercise. Simply read through what I wrote and attempt connecting to the mind of a pre-modern human being.

Additionally, each day this week, practice exercise #3 (p. 77), the focused meditation exercise. Here, unlike a regular meditation, the goal is to focus upon a single event or situation and see what comes up. Feelings, sensations, and images may come up about the situation when you practice these exercises, and they may reveal something important to you about that situation. This exercise is designed to explore a deeper connection to a particular situation. It's an exercise that is similar to the process of remote viewing, which involves seeing things from far away. Practice this exercise once a day during this week.

Now, if you are in this group, you may still have some beliefs about eating, based on media you've consumed, that hinder your intuitive eating experience. If this is the case, write them down if you missed them in exercise #4 (p. 97), on the last day of week 1. Sometimes these beliefs are insidious. We may not be strongly attached to them but they're just there, dictating our choices. Discard them completely until your body approves of them.

As you get into the second week, pay attention to how you're freeing yourself from those beliefs. What actions are you taking to challenge those beliefs? Once you've challenged them, practice exercise #8 (p. 145), "Eating Slow and Silently" with one meal per day. This exercise demands your fullest attention, and I don't recommend doing it with each meal, as you may feel mentally exhausted after a while. The reason why this exercise is recommended for daily practice in the second week instead of the first week is because during the first week, I want you to pay attention to your general satisfaction with what you eat.

But this week, with exercise #8, you will ramp things up a little bit. By chewing your food more thoroughly and being mindful of any and all sensations that arise as you eat, you will possibly receive greater insights. It will be like you're meditating while you're eating. And since meditation is one tool to unlock your intuition, practicing this daily will help you strengthen it.

Lastly, on the last day of this week, evaluate the intuition-blockers in your life, as we did in exercise #5 (p. 106). Look through your answers and evaluate your progress. Are there any factors that you feel are still blocking your intuition? Bring awareness to it and set the attention to relieve the impact of that factor. Don't forget to practice the "Grocery Bonanza" exercise once this week (exercise #9, p. 150).

WEEK 3

This week is the same as week 2: practice the exercises as described above. Since it's important to adjust however, I have some additional tips. Ask yourself what progress you've made, and which areas need the most work. Are you able to understand when you're hungry? Do you know what motivates you to eat? Are you seeing an improvement in any aspect of your wellbeing by eating more intuitively now?

Is there a sticking point? Identify it and work on this sticking point this week. Since it's been two weeks now, you've likely expanded your food memory and developed a palate. Now would be a great time to repeat and refine your methods, as in steps 3 and 4 of *HYMTE* (see chapter 7). Eat new things and some of the same things you've been eating. Keep paying attention to how close your intuitive desire for a food matches how satisfied you are with it afterwards. This is an indicator of how calibrated your intuition is. Remember to practice "Grocery Bonanza" again, but consider practicing it in a different setting this time, such as at a farmer's market.

WEEK 4

This week, I want you to evaluate your progress. At the start of the week, complete exercises 6 (p. 122) and 7 (p. 126) again. Exercise 6 had you list out qualities of foods and what feelings arose with each quality. Exercise 7 is a food-focused meditation, where the goal is to receive sensations about a particular food. You can choose an entire meal here if you'd like to, to study the combinations of foods.

I hope that by now you have a greater sense of clarity in deciding what to eat and can track the foods you eat with after-effects better, to prepare for the day ahead. Practice exercise #1 again (walking meditation in nature) at any time this week, perhaps near the end.

As you go through your day, practice a modification of exercise #3 (p. 77), the focused meditation exercise. Instead of meditating on one single situation, pay attention to the sensations that arise as you observe the happenings of your day. Notice those instantaneous intuitive insights that arise. Those judgments that we often suppress. Bring them to light. Give intuition the microphone. Be guided more and more by these sensations. Try making more decisions off these sensations and decide how you like the consequences.

Instead of recommending specific exercises, this week I want you to focus on intuitive ease: how well you're able to decide what to eat without thinking. The easier it is for you to go from being hungry to deciding what to eat, the better you are at eating intuitively. You know what you want to eat and feel great when you get what you want. This means you're calibrated and have knowledge of how your body operates. Isn't that a gratifying and empowering feeling?

Continue to practice eating slowly. It doesn't have to be done as an exercise. Just take one meal out of your day to eat without distractions and observe the sensations that arise. Tune into your needs. Once this week, practice exercise 6 and 7 again with new foods. By the end of the month, you may have 20-30 foods listed out in exercise 6, with their qualities and how they make you feel. This is good work.

Finally, at the end of the week, read through your answers to the exercises you've completed, especially exercises 4 ("Identifying Your Food Beliefs") and 5 ("Identifying the Intuition Blockers in Your Life"). See what has changed. How is this change going to benefit your health? What more is needed?

Congratulate yourself now and continue to develop your intuition in the months ahead.

10:
Possibility

Food is our common ground, a universal experience.

—JAMES BEARD

INTUITION IS TO SCIENCE as yin is to yang. It's not as forceful and not as glorious as science. Its accomplishments may be just as grand, but they aren't results of conquest and problem-solving. Perhaps the most impressive feats are natural partnerships between science and intuition that arise out of the need for solutions to pressing problems. This would explain why some of the most notable Western minds of the past, Immanuel Kant, Richard Feynman, and Albert Einstein, praised intuition. It's underrated.

Science does provide us with solutions to our health. But what seems fringe, and yet should not be, is that intuition can as well. But how much? Can intuition really improve our health as much as science can? Considering that new technologies may drastically alter the landscape of healthcare in the coming decades, intuition may become even less of an underdog than it is, and more like an invisible blip on our radar in comparison to the behemoth that is biotechnology.

As I've written this, I've asked myself what the possibilities really are for intuition. Just a year ago, I was immersed in a medical program where reductionist science dominated my thinking. I spoke carefully about everything, understanding that there are immense uncertainties in science, and that things always change. Science is just as unpredictable as intuition, but it's also less clear. Transitioning from this background to my current state where I embrace intuition has been interesting, as I now speak with more clarity, confidence, and am less concerned with being incorrect.

But for the scientist, this is anathema. Humility is important, although, arrogance appears to be the norm in many fields. I know that the professors that have had the greatest impact on my own reasoning abilities throughout my education were humble, as they saw the complexity to acquiring knowledge, and that the more one learns, the more there is to learn.

I don't believe that the new confidence I've gained from understanding my intuition leads to a lack of humility at all. It's just a bit surprising in retrospect, as it's a stark contrast with the way I had taught myself to speak, think, and act, in the name of science. I try to always be open to new knowledge and possibilities, but recognizing intuition more and more in my life now, I cannot help but to follow my gut instincts, and have more and more confidence that they will lead me in the right direction.

Thus, I'm curious what your thoughts are regarding the possibility of intuition. For those who are trained to think exactly in the way schools teach science, the concepts in this book may seem off-kilter. But for those who do resonate, what do you think is possible?

I believe the possibilities that may result from applying intuition to our health are just as grand as the possibilities in store for science—in fact, even more so perhaps, as I believe in the stories of medical intuitives; I believe that shamans saw DNA in their ayahuasca visions, and I believe that there are deep truths and mysteries in nature that science has only begun to unearth, and perhaps may never do so.

Closing Thoughts

Every one of the ideas I've shared with you in the previous nine chapters are from my personal experiences with intuition and my attempt to understand science since I started learning about health. These ideas cannot be taught but only shared. You must develop your own personal experiences with eating to guide you in the best direction for your health. If you put some effort into it, you may just discover things you would have never thought possible. Don't go by what anyone says. Go by what you feel from your experience, keeping an open mind to new experiences which you have not had.

I hope this book has given you the fundamentals to understand your eating patterns and habits. With the plethora of diet books on the market that explain *what* to eat, few discuss the how, which comes first. Eating is an intimate experience that is integral to our lives, and when we are disconnected from the process, it can cause malnutrition, stress, and a variety of other problems. Food gives us peace, once we learn to first make peace with food and enjoy it.

If the ideas in this book worked for you, please consider reviewing this book on Amazon. If it didn't work, feel free to let me know there as well; I want to know if this truly worked for you.

Share Your Tips on Connecting to Food

I've created an Instagram account (@hymte_) dedicated to sharing qualitative and intuitive experiences with food. Feel free to add me on there and share your experiences by tagging me in your pictures or by using #hymte as a hashtag. In the near future, there may also be a forum for *HYMTE*. Sign up for the *Stop Being Confused About Health* newsletter on my website to be notified of any upcoming announcements therein.

About Stop Being Confused About Health

After discovering that one of my hairs was gray at the age of 20 (this was after a year of veganism), I realized something was wrong, but didn't know how to stop doing what I was doing. I attribute this premature graying to excessively strenuous weight lifting without adequate recovery, as this has been the largest and most chronic stressor in my life since becoming interested in health.

I started *Stop Being Confused About Health* as a blog to educate readers about the dangers of excessive dieting and exercise. Now, four years later, it's a space where I attempt to share the truth about all things health. My goal is to continue my education and share what I'm learning in the process through writing.

Over there, I discuss various health myths, ancestral health, and aim to promote a balanced way of doing things, while keeping things unfiltered. Check it out at www.stopbeingconfusedabouthealth.com.

References and Notes

[1] Beil K, Hanes D. The influence of urban natural and built environments on physiological and psychological measures of stress- A pilot study. *International Journal of Environmental Research and Public Health*. 2013;10(4):1250-1267.

[2] From the front page of Soylent's website, Soylent is for you if "…you've ever wasted time and energy trying to decide what to eat for lunch, or have been too busy to eat a proper meal…" The product has a 1 year shelf life and does not require refrigeration or preservatives to ensure stability. It is free of animal products, has no cholesterol, and contains only 2g of saturated fat.

[3] Cook JD, Reddy MB. Effect of ascorbic acid intake on nonheme-iron absorption from a complete diet. *American Journal of Clinical Nutrition*. 2001;73(1):93-98.

[4] Teucher B, Olivares M, Cori H. Enhancers of Iron Absorption: Ascorbic Acid and other Organic Acids. *International Journal for Vitamin and Nutrition Research*. 2004;74(6):403-419.

[5] Lynch SR, Cook JD. INTERACTION OF VITAMIN C AND IRON. *Annals of the New York Academy of Sciences*. 1980;355(1 Micronutrient):32-44..

[6] Ioannidis JPA. Why Most Published Research Findings Are False. *PLoS Medicine*. 2005;2(8):e124..

[7] Dr. Duke's Phytochemical and Ethnobotanical Databases. Using this database you can search for a plant and see what its chemical constituents are.

[8] *Curcuma longa*. Dr. Duke's Phytochemical and Ethnobotanical Databases.

[9] United States Department of Agriculture. The Healthy Eating Index. Online.

[10] For more information read "Nutrition and Physical Degeneration" by Weston A. Price, and "Deep Nutrition" by Catherine Shanahan.

[11] Shanahan S, Luke S. Deep Nutrition: Why Your Genes Need Traditional Food. New York, N.Y. Flat Iron Books. 2008. Print.

[12] Sacks FM, Lichtenstein AH, Wu JHY, et al. Dietary Fats and Cardiovascular Disease: A Presidential Advisory From the American Heart Association. *Circulation*. 2017;(Cvd).

[13] Ramsden CE, Zamora D, Majchrzak-Hong S, et al. Re-evaluation of the traditional diet-heart hypothesis: analysis of recovered data from Minnesota Coronary Experiment (1968-73). *British Medical Journal*. 2016;353:i1246.

[14] Saha A. Does Eating Eggs Raise Cholesterol? No, Not According to the Science. *Stop Being Confused About Health*. October, 2017. Online.

[15] Turpeinen O, Karvonen MJ, Pekkarinen M, Miettinen M, Elosuo R, Paavilainen E. Dietary prevention of coronary heart disease: the Finnish Mental Hospital Study. *International Journal of Epidemiology*. 1979;8:99–118.

[16] Burros, M. MARGARINE CHOICES: A GUIDE FOR CONSUMERS. *The New York Times*. 1984.

[17] Geary, KM. Is the American Heart Association a Terrorist Association? *Medium*. June 2017.

[18] Witton K. Phenothiazines and Sudden Death. *Journal of the American Medical Association*. 1965;194(6):679.

[19] Leestma JE, Koenig KL. Sudden Death and Phenothiazines. *Archives of General Psychiatry*. 1968;18(2):137.

[20] Blachly PH. Phenothiazines and Sudden Death. *Journal of the American Medical Association*. 1965;193(7):628.

[21] Seller C, Oosthuizen P. The effects of thioridazine on the QTc interval — cardiovascular safety in a South African setting. *South African Journal of Psychiatry*. 2005;11(2): 46-50.

[22] Wendkos MH. The Significance of Electrocardiographic Changes Produced by Thioridazine. *Journal of New Drugs*. 1964;4(6):322-332.

[23] Thanacoody HKR, Thomas SHL. Tricyclic antidepressant poisoning : cardiovascular toxicity. *Critical Reviews in Toxicology*. 2005;24(3):205-214.

[24] Araujo de Vizcarrondo C, Carrillo de Padilla F, Martín E. Fatty acid composition of beef, pork, and poultry fresh cuts, and some of their processed products. *Archivos Latinoamericanos De Nutrición*. 1998;48(4):354-358.

[25] Food and Nutrition Roundtable. Smart Choices program. Accessed online.

[26] Gordis, L. Epidemiology. Philadelphia. Elsevier Saunders. 2014, pp. 13-14. Print.

[27] Ding M, Bhupathiraju SN, Chen M, van Dam RM, Hu FB. Caffeinated and Decaffeinated Coffee Consumption and Risk of Type 2 Diabetes: A Systematic Review and a Dose-Response Meta-analysis. *Diabetes Care*. 2014;37(2):569-586.

[28] Moisey LL, Robinson LE, Graham TE. Consumption of caffeinated coffee and a high carbohydrate meal affects postprandial metabolism of a subsequent oral glucose tolerance test in young, healthy males. *British Journal of Nutrition*. 2010;103(6):833.

[29] Beinfield H, Korngold E. Between Heaven and Earth: A Guide to Traditional Chinese Medicine. New York. The Random House Publishing Group. 1991. Print.

[30] Saadi HF, Dawodu A, Afandi BO, Zayed R, Benedict S, Nagelkerke N. Efficacy of daily and monthly high-dose calciferol in vitamin D-deficient nulliparous and lactating women. *American Journal of Clinical Nutrition*. 2007;85(6):1565-1571.

[31] Gurd BJ, Giles MD, Bonafiglia JT, et al. Incidence of nonresponse and individual patterns of response following sprint interval training. *Applied Nutrition, Physiology, and Metabolism*. 2016;41(3):229-234. doi:10.1139/apnm-2015-0449.

[32] Pietiläinen KH, Saarni SE, Kaprio J, Rissanen A. Does dieting make you fat? A twin study. *International Journal of Obesity*. 2012;36(3):456-464.

[33] Arcelus J, Mitchell AJ, Wales J, Nielsen S. Mortality Rates in Patients With Anorexia Nervosa and Other Eating Disorders. *Archives of General Psychiatry*. 2011;68(7):724.

[34] Schnorr SL, Candela M, Rampelli S, et al. Gut microbiome of the Hadza hunter-gatherers. *Nature Communications*. 2014;5.

[35] Sutherland C. The Body Knows: How to Tune in to Your Body and Improve Your Health. Carlsbad, CA. Hay House Inc. 2001. Print.

[36] Talbot M. The Holographic Universe: The Revolutionary Theory of Reality. New York, NY. HarperCollins Books. 1992. Print.

[37] Narby J. The Cosmic Serpent: DNA and the Origins of Life. New York. Penguin Putnam Inc. 1998. Print.

[38] Phillips KM, Carlsen MH, Blomhoff R. Total Antioxidant Content of Alternatives to Refined Sugar. *Journal of the American Dietetic Association*. 2009;109(1):64-71.

[39] Johnson RE, Murad MH. Gynecomastia: pathophysiology, evaluation, and management. *Mayo Clin Proceedings*. 2009;84(11):1010-1015.

[40] Biro FM, Lucky AW, Huster GA, Morrison JA. Hormonal studies and physical maturation in adolescent gynecomastia. *Journal of Pediatrics*. 1990;116(3):450-455.

[41] de Ronde W, de Jong FH. Aromatase inhibitors in men: effects and therapeutic options. *Reproductive Biology and Endocrinoly*. 2011;9:93.

[42] 180 Degree Health. Home of Matt Stone and Garret Smith. Online

[43] Vithoulkas, G. A New Model for Health and Disease. Mill Valley, CA. Health and Habitat. Berkeley, CA. North Atlantic Books. 1991. Accessed online.

[44] For further reading on the neurobiology of the reward pathway read "The Compass of Pleasure: How Our Bodies Make Fatty Foods, Orgasm, Exercise, Marijuana, Generosity, Vodka, Learning, and Gambling Feel So Good" by David J. Linden.

[45] Ahmadkhaniha R, Mansouri M, Yunesian M, et al. Association of urinary bisphenol a concentration with type-2 diabetes mellitus. *Journal of Environmental Health Science and Engineering*. 2014;12(1):64.

[46] Achour A, Derouiche A, Barhoumi B, et al. Organochlorine pesticides and polychlorinated biphenyls in human adipose tissue from northern Tunisia: Current extent of contamination and contributions of socio-demographic characteristics and dietary habits. *Environmental Research*. 2017;156(March):635-643.

[47] Nickerson K. Environmental Contaminants in Breast Milk. *Journal of Midwifery & Womens Health*. 2006;51(1):26-34.

[48] Genuis SJ, Birkholz D, Ralitsch M, Thibault N. Human detoxification of perfluorinated compounds. *Public Health*. 2010;124(7):367-375.

[49] Turnbaugh PJ, Ley RE, Mahowald MA, Magrini V, Mardis ER, Gordon JI. An obesity-associated gut microbiome with increased capacity for energy harvest. *Nature*. 2006;444(7122):1027-1031.

[50] Alcock J, Maley CC, Aktipis CA. Is eating behavior manipulated by the gastrointestinal microbiota? Evolutionary pressures and potential mechanisms. *BioEssays*. 2014;36(10):940-949.

32065237R00117

Made in the USA
San Bernardino, CA
10 April 2019